Safety in Healthcare Facilities

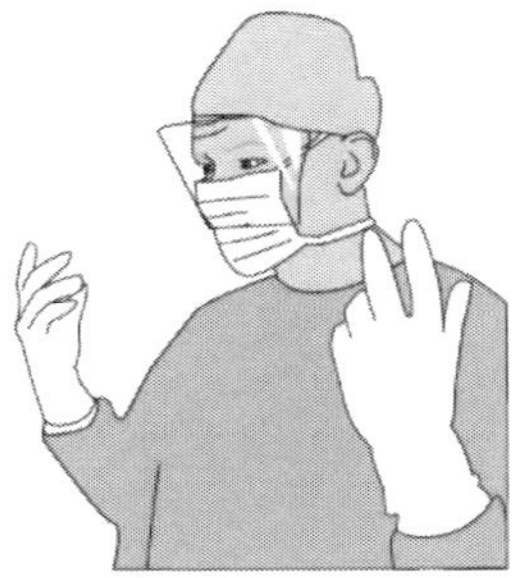

Nicholas Cram

MS, CBET, CHSP
Dominion Biomedical

Selby Holder

CBET

Texas State Technical College Waco

TSTC Publishing

ISBN 978-1-934302-03-3

TSTC Publishing
Texas State Technical College Waco
3801 Campus Drive
Waco, Texas 76705

http://publishing.tstc.edu/

Publisher: Mark Long
Editor: Christopher Wilson
Graphics specialist: Grace Arsiaga
Printing production: Bill Evridge
Illustrations: Jimmy Wisehart

Manufactured in the United States of America

First edition

Table of Contents

Dedication

The authors would like to dedicate this book to our wives Denyce Cram and Tammie Holder. They have been our support systems and our sounding boards on countless nights, dragging us over writer's block and listening to the diatribes common to authors. They have also sacrificed their well deserved "quality time" with the understanding of our desire to contribute to our academic field.

We would also like to thank our students for providing us with a motivation to write a textbook applicable to their career field.

Lastly, we would like to thank our publisher Mark Long. His patience, persistence, encouragement and not-so-subtle prodding have pushed us beyond our own expectations to meet deadlines and produce a textbook of a quality that otherwise would not have been possible.

Nicholas Cram & Selby Holder

Introduction

Every private and public facility and your own home pose safety threats and risks. Many of these potentially harmful conditions within enclosed structures have common linkages, regardless of the type, size or activity within those defined enclosures. Healthcare facilities include all of the potential safety risks of other facilities and have added inherent risks due to the nature of their activities, which are uncommon to any other business or service. Because of the special nature of the activities in a hospital, surgical clinic or nursing home (the business of saving lives and improving the quality of life), there are very strict building codes, standards and regulations that apply specifically to healthcare facilities and the activities that take place within them.

This book will address all of the major safety risks involved in the non-patient care aspects of healthcare facilities. This book is intended to be a textbook for students who require knowledge of safety risks and regulations within a healthcare facility. Typical healthcare careers for which this knowledge is required will be the Vice President of Operations, Vice President of Support Services, Hospital Safety Officer, Director of Plant Operations and Engineering, Director of Clinical Engineering, Biomedical/ Clinical Engineers, and Biomedical Equipment Technicians (BMETs). It is also an ideal handbook for hospital safety committees, inspectors employed by the Joint Commission for Accreditation of Healthcare Organizations and governmental agencies involved in healthcare regulations.

Chapter 1: Defining Safety and Reliability

After reading this chapter, you will have an understanding and applied knowledge of:

- *The definition of safe and safety*
- *The relationship between risk, hazards and safety*
- *The purpose of standard operating procedures and best practices*
- *The differentiation and relationship between safety and reliability*
- *The differentiation between standards and regulations*

The Definition of Safety

Safety involves preventing accidents and/or injuries before they happen. Webster's *New World Dictionary* defines *safe* as "free from damage, danger, etc., secure … having escaped injury, unharmed." Webster's defines *safety* as "… any device for preventing an accident ..." The healthcare environment needs to include standards and regulations, as well as devices intended to prevent an accident or reduce the risk of potential accidents. The first step in creating a safe environment involves awareness of the risks and hazards associated with that environment. With risk and hazard awareness, it is possible to better design healthcare facilities that minimize or avoid certain inherent risks associated with the activities within the building. The best safety mechanism in a healthcare facility is a well trained staff.

The Relationship Between Risk, Hazards and Safety

Every task performed in a healthcare facility involves a certain amount of risk. *Risk* can be defined as the potential or likelihood that an accident will occur. Healthcare facilities have entire departments and/or individuals devoted to risk management. The risk manager in a hospital reviews past accidents or potential accidents and develops guidelines and policies to avoid or prevent future accidents. Risks and hazards in the healthcare arena are always associated with the possibility of improper patient care, loss of quality of life or loss of life itself. A *hazard* can be defined as a dangerous condition or threat associated with certain risks.

A risk manager will attempt to create an environment in the healthcare facility that eliminates or reduces risk in order to avoid unsafe or hazardous situations. The hospital safety committee reviews and establishes facility safety policies.

The Purpose of Standard Operating Procedures and Best Practices

Reducing risks may be accomplished by written policies and procedures that provide instructions for specific tasks. For example, all surgical procedures must be performed with sterile instruments. The instructions on proper sterilization of the surgical instruments are provided by a set of policies or standards. If the policies for instrument sterilization are always followed, the risk of infection during surgery is reduced. Policies and procedures may be developed and enforced by individual healthcare facilities. Generally, industry standards are adopted as the policy or set of instructions for specific tasks performed in daily routines of the healthcare facility. Standards and regulations provide a means of defining specific steps or procedures that must or should be enforced when certain tasks or activities are performed.

Standards are suggested practices adopted by industry in order to reduce or eliminate risks associated with tasks and activities. Sometimes these standards are known as *best practices.* Best practices are policies used repeatedly that provide the best results for a given task or procedure. In addition to industry standards and regulations, healthcare facilities will also adopt *standard operating procedures* (SOPs), which are specific to their facility. These SOPs are a result of previous hazardous or high risk experiences that have occurred in their facility or other facilities. These SOPs are also known as best practices. Best practices are definitive and proven methods or processes used in other industries with exceptional results. Best practices and SOPs are intended to provide the facility with a more efficient, reduced hazard and lower risk environment.

The Differentiation Between Standards and Regulations

There are standards bodies in every profession that develop written procedures recognized and adopted by the industry. Standards bodies do not have the authority to enforce the written procedures they recommend. Healthcare facilities oversee and enforce standards internally in order to reduce risk and improve overall safety of the patients, staff and visitors. Regulations are laws passed by the state or federal government that require certain procedures be followed for specific tasks, designs or activities. Regulations are enforceable by the authorities governing the activity of the regulation. The Food and Drug Administration (FDA), a federal government agency, has the authority granted by the Congress of the United States to remove certain medical devices from a healthcare facility if the device fails to meet certain FDA regulations. These regulations are laws passed by the Congress of the United States. State health departments have the authority to require certain policies be enforced in healthcare facilities located in their state based on laws passed by state legislative bodies.

The purpose of regulations and standards in healthcare is to reduce potential hazards and the risks associated with those hazards. Standards and regulations apply to the technology within a healthcare facility, as well as the design and activity of the healthcare facility. All healthcare personnel must have an appreciation of the importance of standards and regulations specific to their area of responsibility. The processes within a healthcare facility are interrelated. An unsafe condition in any area of the healthcare facility could have potentially hazardous effects on the patient care aspect in other areas of the healthcare facility.

The Differentiation and Relationship Between Safety and Reliability

The safety aspect of technology and the devices associated with technology require an understanding of failure and reliability. *Failure* can be defined as the inability to perform a function as expected. *Reliability* can be defined as the likelihood that a device, process or system will fail. As seen from the definitions of reliability and failure, they are directly related to risk and hazard. If a device, process or system fails in a healthcare facility, there is an increased risk to the patient. Failures create hazards. Hazards increase risks. Maintenance and repair of the technology within a healthcare facility has a direct relationship to the safety of the facility due to hazards created by failure of technology.

Glossary of Terms

Best practices: policies that have been used repeatedly that provide the best results for a given task or procedure.

Failure: the inability to perform a function as expected.

Hazard: a dangerous condition or threat associated with certain risks.

Regulations: laws passed by state or federal government that require certain procedures be followed for specific tasks, designs or activities. Regulations are enforceable by the authorities governing the activity of the regulation.

Reliability: the likelihood that a device, process or system will fail.

Risk: the potential or likelihood that an accident will occur.

Safe: being away from damage or harm; escaping injury.

Safety: involves preventing accidents and/or injuries before they happen.

Standard operating procedures (SOPs): standards adopted by healthcare facilities, which are specific to their facility. These SOPs are a result of previous hazardous or high risk experiences that have occurred in their facility or other facilities.

Chapter 1 Review Questions

Name____

Date____

1) Explain how risk, hazards, and safety are related, but also how each term has a different meaning.

2) Why are standards important?

3) Why are regulations important?

4) Explain the difference between a standard and a regulation.

5) How are *best practices* developed?

6) What is the relationship between *standard operating procedures* (SOP) and *best practices*?

7) When might an SOP and a *best practice* be the same?

Chapter 2: Regulatory Agencies and Standards Bodies

After reading this chapter you will have an understanding and applied knowledge of:

- *The role and identification of healthcare safety standards bodies*
- *The role and identification of healthcare safety regulatory bodies*
- *The role of the Occupational Safety Health Administration in healthcare safety*
- *The role of state health departments in healthcare safety*
- *The role and activities of the hospital safety committee*
- *The role of the Joint Commission on Accreditation of Healthcare Organizations related to hospital and patient safety*
- *The relationship of the Joint Commission on Accreditation of Healthcare Organizations to the hospital safety committee*

Codes, Standards and Regulations

Codes, standards and regulations are becoming increasingly important in the healthcare environment. The purpose of these three types of guidelines is to protect the employees and patients within healthcare facilities.

A *code* is defined as a "systematic statement of a body of law" or "a system of principles or rules" in Webster's *Ninth New Collegiate Dictionary*. Codes within a healthcare facility consist of a collection of guidelines that have been accepted by numerous organizations. These organizations are normally made up of volunteers within the different areas and who are experts on the different topics and areas they govern. Some examples of these organizations are the National Fire Protection Association, Association for the Advancement of Medical Instrumentation and the American National Standards Institute. These organizations are the backbone of many federal, state and local guidelines that are required in healthcare facilities today.

Standards, on the other hand, are the specific documents used to establish a specific level of performance for a piece of equipment, establish uniform testing methods for equipment, establish procedures for material handling, and establish guidelines for specific procedures. The guidelines can be made up within the healthcare facility by the safety committee or be taken from governmental or standards bodies. There are three types of standards used today within the United States: voluntary, mandatory and proprietary.

Voluntary standards are normally defined as those set by manufacturers or providers of specific equipment or supplies within a facility. These standards are derived from numerous public reviews and comments on specific areas and topics. They are usually the direct result of these committees and not from special interest groups.

Mandatory standards are those that are required by law. Some examples include guidelines and regulations published by the Food and Drug Administration, the Occupational Safety and Health Administration, and the Federal Communication Commission.

Proprietary standards are normally developed and used in specific industries or by specific membership associations. Some examples of these standards would be those used by the American Association of Blood Banks. These standards are set to regulate the storage and handling of blood products within healthcare facilities. Although these standards are specific to an area of the hospital or industry, they are sometimes adopted by governmental agencies and put into law.

Regulations are the rules or laws that are adopted by the different enforcement agencies within a specific area. Healthcare facilities must follow these regulations under penalty of law. Throughout the years many codes and standards from the different standard bodies have been adopted by local and state law enforcement.

Standards Bodies

The National Fire Protection Association

As mentioned in chapter one, standards bodies are important to industry for development of uniform practices adopted as a "normal" everyday practice within the facility. In healthcare, the National Fire Protection Association (NFPA) provides standards on a number of practices, including life safety, electrical facility standards and medical device electrical and electronic standards. The NFPA is a voluntary, nonprofit organization with an open membership to individuals and organizations interested in promoting fire safety. The mission of the international nonprofit NFPA is to reduce the worldwide burden of fire and other hazards on the quality of life by providing and advocating consensus codes and standards, research, training, and education.

The 300 codes produced by the NFPA influence every building, process, service, design and installation in the U.S. as well as many other countries. The standards that are published by the NFPA have been developed through an organization of knowledgeable individuals and are made available for public review prior to being adopted. This formal process allows these standards to be considered a "national consensus standard." For these standards to become known as "American National Standards," they must first be recognized and adopted by the American National Standards Institute (ANSI). ANSI coordinates all the standards developed by public and private organizations to help eliminate any inconsistencies or redundancies.

These standards are reviewed and updated on a three-year cycle. The accrediting body for your facility will determine which volume and/or year that is relevant for your facility. In the healthcare environment, there are three main volumes or codes that medical personnel should be very familiar with:

NFPA-70 *National Electrical Code*

NFPA-99 *Standard for Healthcare Facilities*

NFPA-101 *Life Safety Code*

NFPA-70

The National Electrical Code is the most predominant volume used by electricians and maintenance personnel. This volume gives specific regulations for individuals in the areas of wire size, length, voltage and current draws that are allowable in the healthcare facilities. This volume would be referenced when the need for additional power is required, or during installation, construction or remodeling of a specific area within a hospital.

NFPA-99

Biomedical and clinical engineers use these standards for healthcare facilities. This volume contains information on electrical systems, gas and vacuum systems, environmental systems, electrical equipment, gas equipment, laboratories, hospital requirements, ambulatory healthcare requirements, safe use of high-frequency electricity in healthcare facilities and flammable anesthetizing locations. This is the most referenced volume when determining the requirements or testing intervals for medical devices.

NFPA-101

Life Safety Code is used by engineering and maintenance personnel to give them guidance in the area of building safety in the healthcare environment. Although the NFPA is not a federal organization, ANSI has accepted and approved their standards. Also, OSHA (Occupational Safety and Health Administration) uses their standards to enforce laws dealing with employee workplace safety. Cities, counties, states and other organizations that have jurisdiction in your area also frequently require these guidelines and regulations.

Association for the Advancement of Medical Instrumentation

The Association for the Advancement of Medical Instrumentation (AAMI) was founded in 1967. The mission of its 6,000+ members is to work together to increase the understanding and beneficial use of medical instrumentation. They are the resource for industry and governmental agencies for national and international standards. In conjunction with ANSI, they have developed and managed the many different standards used today within healthcare facilities. This organization was the first to certify individuals in the biomedical, radiological and laboratory fields. In recent years this organization has turned this service over to the International Certification Commission (ICC). AAMI holds annual meetings to review and discuss recent trends and advancements in the medical field. They also provide continuing education, and publish technical documents, periodicals, books, and software, and hold conferences to allow their members to strive to be the most informed in their specific area.

American National Standards Institute

The American National Standards Institute (ANSI) is the coordinator of the U.S. voluntary standardization system. Through its committees and working groups, the institute facilitates the development of American standards. This organization has worked in conjunction with OSHA to provide standards for workplace safety. This organization also provides standards for electronic and test devices used in medical facilities.

Regulatory Bodies

Occupational Safety and Health Administration

The Occupational Safety and Health Administration (OSHA) is a governmental organization whose mission is to ensure the safety and health of America's workers by setting and enforcing standards; providing training, outreach and education; establishing partnerships; and encouraging continual improvement in workplace safety and health. Their standards can be seen in every facet of the workplace, such as wet floor signage, exit signage and many other types of signs and processes that help to reduce accidents and prevent injury to employees.

Food and Drug Administration

The Food and Drug Administration (FDA) is a governmental organization whose mission is to protect the public health by assuring the safety, efficacy and security of human and veterinary drugs, biological products, medical devices, the nation's food supply, cosmetics, and products that emit radiation. The FDA is also responsible for advancing public health by helping to speed innovations that make medicines and foods more effective, safer, and more affordable, and helping the public get the accurate, science-based information they need to use medicines and foods to improve their health.

They are the federal organization that approves all medical devices, procedures and medicines used in medical facilities. As with the previously listed, medical equipment must go through the 510K process. This is the trial process to verify the operation and safety of all medical devices. All medical devices that are used in the U.S. must go through this process before they can be sold to medical facilities.

State Health Departments

The local state health departments within many states are the governing bodies for healthcare facilities. They are the agency that inspects and accredits facilities to operate within their state. The guidelines used for these inspections may be only a minimum standard. If your facility is accredited by other organizations, such as Association of American Blood Banks (AABB), College of American Pathologists (CAP), Joint Commission of the Accreditation of Healthcare Organizations (JCAHO), etc., there may be more stringent guidelines or regulations that your facility may have to meet. The administration within the facility should know the different guidelines and standards that need to be met and can put in place the appropriate education to meet them.

Centers for Disease Control and Prevention (CDC)

The Centers for Disease Control and Prevention (CDC) is a federal agency within the Department of Health and Human Services. There are four major coordinating centers that respond to health threats and provide health information to the public and healthcare professionals. A wealth of information can be obtained from its Web site at www.cdc.gov.

The Coordinating Center for Environmental Health and Injury Prevention consists of two branches. The National Center for Environmental Health/Agency for Toxic Substances and Disease Registry (NCEH-ATSDR) has the responsibility for providing public information concerning interventions to prevent death, injury or disease from poisons, microbial contaminations and other toxins that are released into the environment. The National Center for Injury Prevention and Control (NCIPC) has the responsibility to prevent death and disability from hazards not related to occupation.

The Coordinating Center for Health Information and Services has three service branches. The National Center for Health Statistics (NCHS) provides information as a guideline for healthcare policy makers. The National Center for Public Health Informatics (NCPHI) provides applications in information technology that can be of use in the public health environment. The National Center for Health Marketing (NCHM) provides information and applications in health marketing science to benefit public health.

The Coordinating Center for Health Promotion has three service branches. The National Center on Birth Defects and Developmental Disabilities (NCBDDD) has a responsibility for providing information and guidance for prevention of birth defects, developmental disabilities and improving the health and quality of life for people with disabilities. The National Center for Chronic Disease Prevention and Health Promotion (NCCDPHP) provides information and guidance to prevent premature death from disabilities and promotes the adoption of healthy individual activities. The Office of Genomics and Disease Prevention is a relatively new service branch resulting from the Human Genome Project. This CDC service branch coordinates information obtained from genomic research and applies it to improve health and disease prevention.

The Coordinating Center for Infectious Diseases is one of the original core services of the CDC. There are six service branches involved in infectious disease control and prevention. The National Center for Infectious Diseases (NCID) has an international focus on the prevention of illness, disability or death caused by infectious diseases. The National Immunization Program (NIP) coordinates the availability and use of vaccines for children and adults. The National Center for HIV, STD and TB Prevention (NCHSTP) provides direction and information for the intervention and control of immunodeficiency virus infection, sexually transmitted diseases and tuberculosis. The Coordinating Office for Global Health is active internationally in the coordination of national CDC policies and activities and those of the international community.

The Coordinating Office for Terrorism Preparedness and Emergency Responses provides a strategic plan for regional and local health centers to prepare them as first responders. The National Institute for Occupational Safety and Health (NIOSH) is responsible for workplace safety and health. NIOSH provides information on hazard prevention in the workplace and responds to all issues involving employee injury and health.

Joint Commission on Accreditation of Healthcare Organizations

The Joint Commission on Accreditation of Healthcare Organizations (JCAHO) is a voluntary accreditation organization. They are specific to acute care, extended care, ambulatory care and home care facilities. They are a nonprofit organization that surveys hospitals every three years on a fee-for-service basis. This organization surveys every process in the facility from documentation to everyday operation of all aspects of the facilities. This accreditation is necessary to maintain "deemed" status for reimbursement by Medicare and other federally funded programs. In addition to federally funded programs, medical and nursing training programs can only be implemented in accredited facilities. Over the past few years, JCAHO has changed some if its survey tactics. To ensure the compliance of standards throughout the facility, they have started surveying facilities on weekends and in the evening to ensure that all staff work within the standards set by the organization. They have also instituted unannounced visits on facilities that have had a recent sentinel event (any event that has caused serious injury or death to a patient).

Hospital Safety Committees

The hospital safety committee is an internal (within the organization) body that serves as a major component of the Joint Commission on Accreditation of Healthcare Organizations. All accidents and high risk practices are reviewed by the safety committee. The purpose of the hospital safety committee is to assess risk, and enforce and propose Standard Operating Procedures in order to reduce hazards within the healthcare facility. The members of the hospital safety committee are usually directors of major clinical departments such as nursing, dietary, physical therapy and imaging. Non-clinical members of the safety committee include plant operations, maintenance and engineering, housekeeping and security. The hospital safety officer presides over the meetings and sets the agenda.

The clinical/biomedical engineering department is a critical member of the safety committee with responsibilities for all medical equipment errors that pose risks or are involved in patient injury or death. Depending on the roles within the hospital, the clinical/biomedical engineering department may be considered either a clinical or non-clinical department.

The JCAHO has seven core elements that are part of the "Environment of Care" concept, which every hospital safety committee utilizes as a baseline for record keeping and standard operating procedures related to safety issues. The safety components of the Environment of Care include:

1) Safety management

2) Security management

3) Hazardous materials and wastes

4) Life safety

5) Emergency preparedness (bioterrorist threats, internal and external disasters)

6) Medical equipment management

7) Utility management

Glossary of Terms

American National Standards Institute (ANSI): the coordinator of the U.S. voluntary standardization system. Through its committees and working groups, the institute facilitates the development of American standards. This organization has worked in conjunction with OSHA (Occupational Safety and Health Administration) to provide standards for workplace safety. This organization also provides standards for electronic and tests devices used in medical facilities.

Association for the Advancement of Medical Instrumentation (AAMI): founded in 1967, its mission is to increase the understanding and beneficial use of medical instrumentation. It is the resource for industry and governmental agencies for national and international standards.

Centers for Disease Control and Prevention (CDC): The CDC is a federal agency within the Department of Health and Human Services. There are four major coordinating centers that respond to health threats and provide health information to the public and healthcare professionals.

Code: a "systematic statement of a body of law" or "a system of principles or rules."

Food and Drug Administration (FDA): is a governmental organization whose mission is to protect the public health by assuring the safety, efficacy and security of human and veterinary drugs, biological products, medical devices, the nation's food supply, cosmetics, and products that emit radiation.

Hospital safety committee: an internal (within the organization) body that serves as a major component of the Joint Commission on Accreditation of Healthcare Organizations. All accidents and high risk practices are reviewed by the safety committee. The purpose of the hospital safety committee is to assess risk, enforce and propose Standard Operating Procedures in order to reduce hazards within the healthcare facility.

Joint Commission on Accreditation of Healthcare Organizations (JCAHO): a voluntary accreditation organization. It is specific to acute care, extended care, ambulatory care, and home care facilities. It is a nonprofit organization that surveys hospitals every three years on a fee-for-service basis. This organization surveys every process in the facility from documentation to everyday operation of all aspects of the facilities. The hospital safety committee provides JCAHO with documentation of the safety activities within the hospital. The hospital safety committee is also responsible for implementing the elements of the Environment of Care, which is the core of JCAHO's safety oversight mission.

The National Fire Protection Association (NFPA): a voluntary, nonprofit, international organization with an open membership to individuals and organizations interested in promoting fire safety. The NFPA mission is to reduce the worldwide burden of fire and other hazards on the quality of life by providing and advocating consensus codes and standards, research, training and education.

NFPA-70 National Electrical Code: the most predominantly used volume by electricians and maintenance personnel. This volume gives specific regulations for individuals in the areas of wire size, length, voltage and current draws that are allowable in the healthcare facilities. This volume would be referenced when the need for additional power is required, or during installation or remodeling of a specific area within a hospital.

NFPA-99 Standard for Healthcare Facilities: contains information on electrical systems, gas and vacuum systems, environmental systems, electrical equipment, gas equipment, laboratories, hospital requirements, ambulatory healthcare requirements, safe use of high-frequency electricity in healthcare facilities and flammable anesthetizing locations. This is the most referenced volume when determining the requirements or testing intervals for medical devices. This volume is used extensively by biomedical and clinical engineers for standards related to healthcare facilities.

NFPA-101 Life Safety Code: used by engineering and maintenance personnel to give them guidance in the area of building safety in the healthcare environment.

Occupational Safety and Health Administration (OSHA): a governmental organization whose mission is to ensure the safety and health of America's workers by setting and enforcing standards; providing training, outreach and education; establishing partnerships; and encouraging continual improvement in workplace safety and health.

Regulations: the rules or laws adopted by different enforcement agencies withing a specific area.

Sentinel event: an unexpected occurrence involving death or serious physical/psychological injury.

Standards: the specific documents that are used to try to establish a specific level of performance for a piece of equipment, establish uniform testing methods for equipment, procedures for material handling, and guidelines for specific procedures.

State health departments: the local state health departments within many states are the governing bodies for healthcare facilities. They are the agency that inspects and accredits facilities to operate within their state.

Voluntary standards: those procedures set by manufacturers or providers of specific equipment or supplies within a facility.

Chapter 2 Review Questions

Name____________________________________

Date_____________________________________

1) Explain the differences and similarities in the roles of the State Health Department and the Occupational Safety and Health Administration.

2) Why is the Hospital Safety Committee the most important safety body within a hospital?

3) What is the relationship between the Hospital Safety Committee and the JCAHO?

4) Under what circumstances might a hospital require the expertise of the Centers for Disease Control and Prevention?

5) What branch of the CDC is responsible for bioterrorist protection and response?

6) Which volume of the NFPA contains information relating to healthcare facilities?

7) Which institute facilitates the development of American standards in conjunction with the Occupational Safety and Health Administration?

8) What is the purpose of the Association for the Advancement of Medical Instrumentation?

9) What is the mission of the Food and Drug Administration?

10) What is the difference between a standard and a code?

Chapter 3: Personal Protective Equipment and Disease Prevention

After reading this chapter, you will have an understanding and applied knowledge of:

- *Proper use of Personal Protective Equipment (PPE)*
- *Identifying and understanding how diseases are transmitted (antibiotic resistance)*
- *Identifying and understanding the hazards and risks involved with blood-borne and airborne pathogens*
- *Identifying and understanding the hazards and risks involved with contact pathogens*
- *The role and activities of the hospital infection control nurse*
- *The purpose of tuberculosis testing and vaccines*

Personal Protective Equipment (PPE)

Hospitals contain a myriad of hazards related to physical, chemical, radiological and microbial risks. In order to safely work in this environment, special procedures and special equipment have been developed. This special equipment is known as Personal Protective Equipment (PPE). The PPE is selected, depending on the hazard you may encounter in a particular work environment. In general, protective equipment is designed to eliminate risks to certain parts of the body. For example, latex gloves provide protection to the hands from contact exposure to chemicals and microbes. Technicians who operate or maintain medical equipment that is exposed to body fluids should always wear gloves.

Equipment may appear to be free of hazards but is not. Dried blood containing pathogens (disease causing organisms) may not be visible but a single organism the size of the head of a pin may cause diseases that are incurable. Debris, mildew, mold and contaminated water are other hazards that may be present in disaster situations. PPE must be available for every hazard that may be encountered.

Figure 3.01 *Gloves:* protect the hands from contact exposure and spread of microbes.

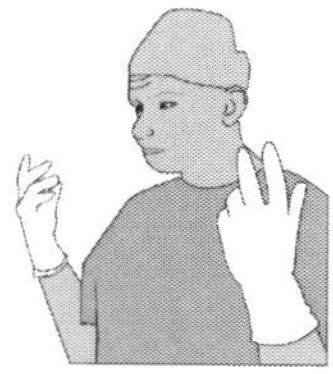

Mask: protects the respiratory system from inhaling airborne contaminants.

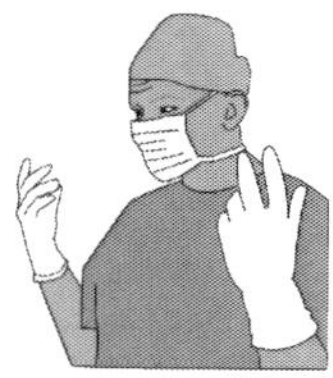

Gowns: protect the torso of the body from spills containing radioactive, caustic, and body fluid hazards.

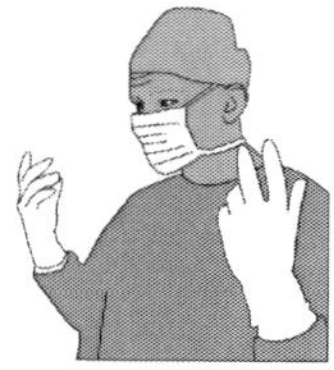

Eye Shield: protects the face and eyes from spills containing radioactive, caustic, and body fluid hazards.

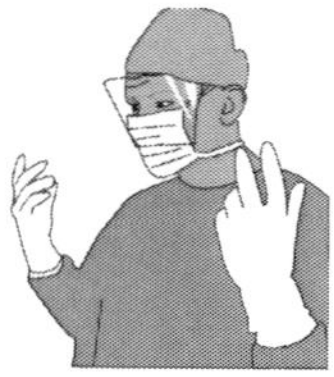

Rubber Boots: protect your footwear from spreading contamination to other parts of your body and to other areas of the hospital.

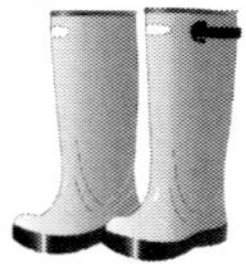

Disease Vectors

People are admitted to hospitals and health centers for a variety of illnesses and medical conditions. Each person entering a hospital has the potential to bring bacteria and viruses, toxic compounds and allergens with them. This includes the patients, guests and staff. Surgical and clinical laboratory departments have the highest risk of spreading contaminants to people throughout the hospital. Personnel working in these areas take special classes to understand what hazards are present and how to protect themselves and their fellow workers.

Diseases and contaminants are spread by the following methods, known as *vectors*:

1) Contact (touching a contaminated item or surface)

2) Airborne (inhaling a contaminated substance or microbe)

3) Blood-borne (physical contact or sprayed droplets of blood that contain microbes)

4) Ingestion (contaminated food and water)

If proper precautions are not taken and PPE is not used, a person exposed to a hazard or infected with a disease may spread this hazard or disease to another person or groups of people.

Antibiotic Resistance

Antibiotics have been a miracle cure for these hazards and microbial diseases since the 1940s. Unfortunately, overuse and misuse of antibiotics has resulted in what are known as "super bugs." These super bugs are not sensitive to the antibiotics and create a serious threat to treatment of several diseases. This lack of sensitivity by super bugs is known as antibiotic resistance. Common resistant organisms are methicillin resistant staphylococcus aureus (MRSA) and vancomycin resistant staphylococcus aureus (VRSA).

Figure 3.02

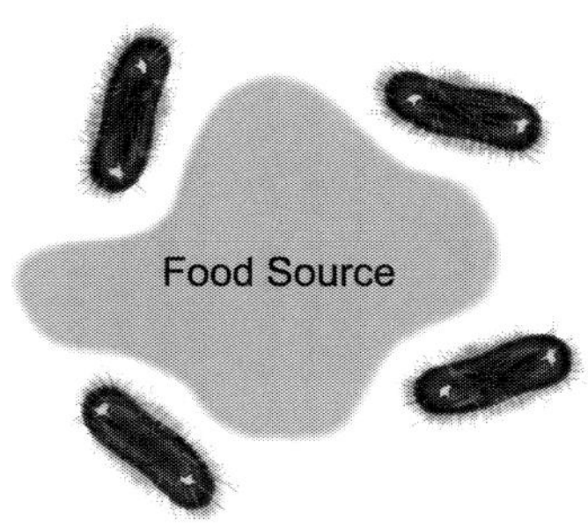

Blood-borne and Airborne Pathogens

Blood-borne pathogens are disease-causing microbes that have spread into a person's bloodstream. Surgical procedures, drawing blood for testing samples and open wounds allow blood from infected patients to create a pathway (soaking on sheets, drops on the floor or furniture) that will spread the pathogen by contact. Dried blood containing viruses such as the human immunodeficiency virus (HIV) can survive for several days on a countertop or other surface. Any person who comes into contact with the pathogen containing dried blood may become infected.

Airborne pathogens are spread by coughing or sneezing. Tiny droplets are released into the air. The tuberculosis (TB) pathogen is so small that it may ride on dust particles in the air and remain there for up to three days. Anyone entering the same room containing the TB "hitchhiker" has a risk of inhaling the pathogen and becoming infected. Patients with known cases of TB will be placed in an isolation room. Isolation rooms have "negative pressure" balance in the airflow into and out of the room. This means that as you enter an isolation room, the outside air from the hallway is sucked into the room. This prevents the airborne pathogen from escaping into the hallway. A special personally fitted mask/respirator must be worn when entering an isolation room. The infection control nurse in each healthcare facility will check your mask to ensure that there are no leaks and the seal of the mask is secure.

Figure 3.03

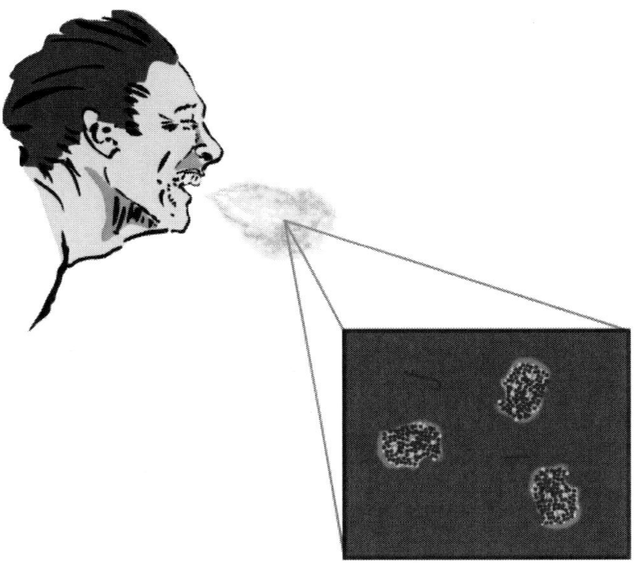

Contact Pathogens

Contact pathogens create the most frequent type of disease-spreading mechanism in and out of the hospital. Hand washing is the single most effective method of preventing exposure to contact pathogens. The clinical lab, operating room and intensive care unit (ICU) have the highest risk of exposure to contact pathogens. A healthcare professional should always assume that a device is contaminated and wear appropriate PPE. Wash your hands after contact with any surface that may have been exposed to a contact pathogen. A common source of contact pathogens are elevator buttons and door knobs. Some hospital employees wear gloves to protect themselves from contact pathogens but do not remove them when leaving the area of possible exposure. These healthcare workers are now part of the disease-spreading process. Anything they touch with their gloves will become a possible source of contact pathogens. Remember, always remove your gloves after you are no longer in danger of contact pathogen exposure. You should never walk around the hospital wearing your gloves.

Figure 3.04

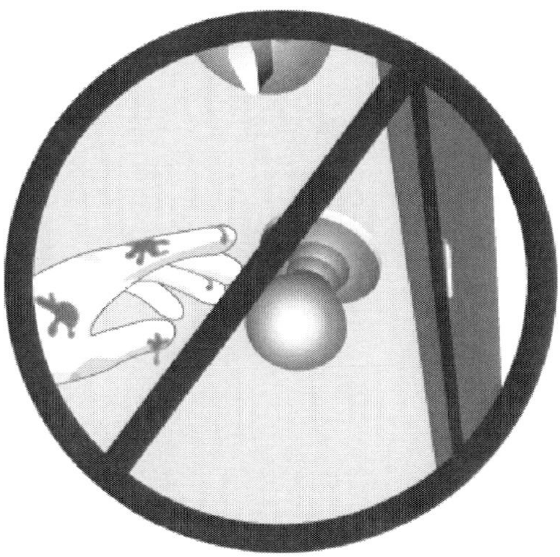

The Hospital Infection Control Nurse

If there is reason to believe that hospital personnel and visitors may become exposed to a pathogen, the infection control nurse has the authority to close off certain parts of the hospital. The infection control nurse also reviews antibiotic treatment therapies. If a biohazard alert is reported from the CDC or local public health officer, the hospital infection control nurse is a key figure in organizing the proper response for the hospital personnel.

Tuberculosis and Hepatitis

Tuberculosis (TB) is a mycobacterium that enters the body through the respiratory system. It lodges in the alveoli sacs of the lungs and may remain dormant until the body's defense system (immune system) becomes weakened. The TB bacterium destroys the tiny alveoli sacs and limits the amount of oxygen that can enter the blood stream. It is also characterized by a persistent cough.

Inside the hospital environment, TB can spread rapidly. It is a threat to all hospital employees and guests. As a precaution, all hospital staff are given a subcutaneous (under the skin) injection of live TB in order to detect the presence of the mycobacterium. This injection does not protect you from TB infection. The purpose of the injection is to determine if you have been exposed to TB. If your test is positive (a red ring-bump remaining on your arm 72 hours after injection), then an X-ray of your lungs will be taken as a positive identification of TB infection. Dark spots on your lungs appearing on the X-ray indicate a positive diagnosis of TB infection.

Hepatitis is a virus that attacks the liver cells. It is a blood-borne pathogen. It may produce an excess of biliruben in the blood, which causes the skin to appear yellow or "jaundiced." A vaccine is injected in a series of three shots over three months to protect healthcare workers from becoming infected with hepatitis.

Glossary of Terms

Antibiotic resistance (super bugs): microbes that lack sensitivity to antibiotics. Caused by overuse and misuse of antibiotics. Common resistant organisms are methicillin resistant staphylococcus aureus (MRSA) and vancomycin resistant staphylococcus aureus (VRSA).

Blood-borne pathogens: disease causing microbes that have spread into a person's blood stream.

Diseases vectors: methods of spreading disease:

1) Contact (touching a contaminated item or surface)

2) Airborne (inhaling a contaminated substance or microbe)

3) Blood-borne (physical contact or sprayed droplets of blood that contain microbes)

4) Ingestion (food and water)

Contact pathogens: surgical procedures, drawing blood for testing samples and open wounds allow blood from infected patients to create a pathway (soaking on sheets, drops on the floor or furniture) that will spread contact with the infected surface.

Infection control nurse: a nurse with specialized training in microbiology and epidemiology. Duties of the infection control nurse include the containment and treatment of infections in the hospital, training and attentiveness to pathogenic hazards. The infection control nurse is also a member of the hospital safety committee.

Personal Protective Equipment (PPE): special equipment to protect healthcare workers from hazards related to physical, chemical, radiological and microbial risks.

Chapter 3 Review Questions

Name________________________________

Date________________________________

1) Explain four disease vectors that could expose you to a pathogen.

2) What is the single most effective means to prevent the spread of disease in a hospital?

3) Explain the role and activities of the infection control nurse.

4) What areas of the hospital have the highest risk for blood-borne pathogen contact?

5) Why should you wear gloves when entering a patient's room?

6) What PPE would be required to enter an isolation room known to have an active TB patient?

7) How do bacteria and viruses become resistant to antibiotics?

8) Why is it important that your personal respirator mask has a tight seal?

9) Explain why it is a health hazard to continue to wear disposable gloves after leaving a contaminated area.

10) If you are walking down a hallway in the hospital and notice a blood spill on the floor, what actions should you take?

Chapter 4: Electric Shock and Industrial Safety Systems

After completing this chapter you will have an understanding and applied knowledge of:

- *Electrical shock hazards associated with the repair of electronic components*
- *Electrical monitoring and protection devices used to create a safe environment wherever electronic devices may be used*
- *The one-hand rule for personal protection from shock hazards, when repairing electronic components*
- *The skin effect of electrical current*
- *Voltage potentials*
- *National Fire Protection Association Section 99 electrical safety requirements for medical devices*
- *The purpose of grounding*

Safety Practices

Voltage Potentials

Voltage potentials are created when the voltage at one point is higher than a voltage at another point, with respect to the reference point or ground. Potential differences in voltage due to variable grounding sources create a unique hazard with electronic devices. The common reference point for a voltage potential may be the facility electrical conduit, the facility plumbing fixtures, the device associated with patient or consumer use, or other people in contact with any combination of the above reference points.

Voltage potentials can be created during the renovation or new construction associated with the same electrical path. Old wiring that has become corroded or worn wiring insulation can also be sources of voltage potentials. Any of these combinations cause a difference in the resistance of the current path.

Because of the potential harm related to electric shock, special equipment and facility design consideration and monitoring instrumentation are required for both electronic devices and the facilities where they are located. The best electrical safety system in a facility is a well trained staff.

Safety: The One-Hand Rule

Due to the many hazards related to repair and maintenance of medical and consumer electronic devices, special safety rules such as the *one-hand rule* have been developed.

The premise of the one-hand rule states that when inserting tools or touching any component of a device, one hand should be held purposefully away from the device so that only the tool-holding hand will have a possibility of contact with electric current. This prevents the creation of a completed circuit across the chest and heart, and returning through the chassis (conductive case) of the device.

Figure 4.01

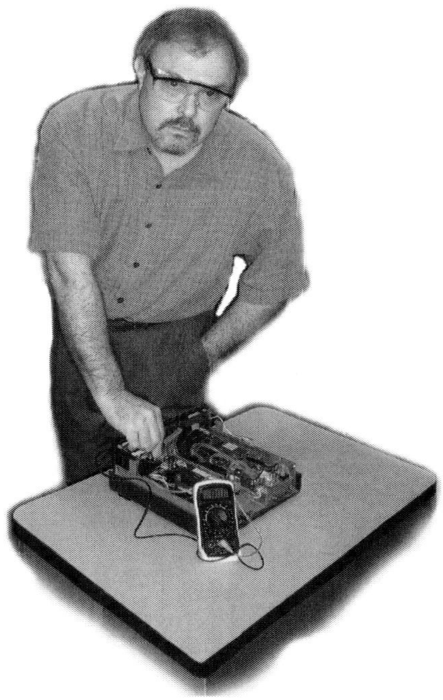

Patients are most susceptible to voltage potentials and current leakage when there is a nonstandard method of common grounding. All medical devices, electric beds, and other electronic devices (e.g. televisions) in a common room should have a common grounding reference. This is especially important if housekeeping enters a patient room with a high-voltage device such as a buffer, or in circumstances in which portable high-voltage medical devices such as ultrasound or X-ray units are used at the patient's bedside. If a voltage potential develops and the metal portion of a bed becomes part of the circuit, microshock (a shock across the heart) could occur.

Figure 4.02

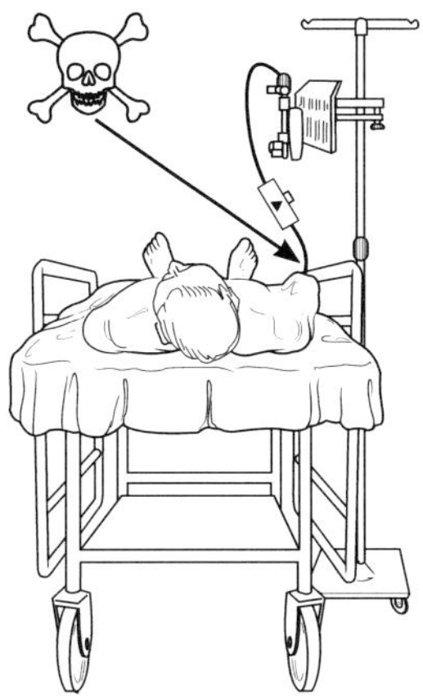

A 10μV voltage potential could cause cardioversion.

Figure 4.03

Common power bus

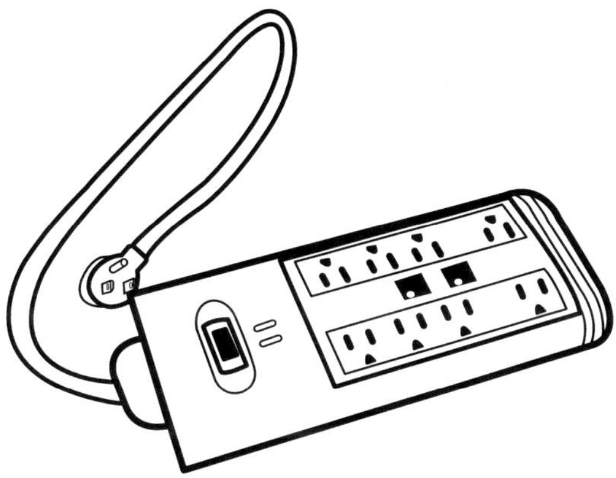

Multiple connections to power buses can create potential safety hazards from power cords crossing in the same area and also as a fire hazard due to high currents flowing into one circuit.

Intravenous (IV) lines represent one of the most serious hazards of leakage current and grounding potentials in the health care environment. An IV line provides a direct path to the heart. A current of 10μA can cause cardioversion (interruption of the heartbeat) if leakage current enters the intravenous catheter site.

The electrical panel should accommodate the required current and the grounding of all receptacles should have a common reference. A visitor, physician, or nurse can provide a source of electrical continuity between any bedside device and the bed railing or patient if the grounding is not unified.

Macroshock and Microshock

Electric Shock

Electric shock is an unwelcome and avoidable physiological response to current. Electrical stimulation may cause a cellular depolarization due to a change in membrane potential by approximately 20%. The result can range from muscle contraction, injury or death from cardiac failure or respiratory failure.

Macroshock is a physiological response to a current applied to the surface of the body (e.g. hand) that produces an electrical shock resulting in an unwelcome and avoidable physiological response to current and unwanted and unnecessary stimulation, muscle contractions or tissue damage.

Microshock is a physiological response to current applied to the surface of the heart that results in electrical shock as an unwelcome or avoidable physiological response to current and unwanted or unnecessary stimulation, muscle contractions, or tissue damage. In contrast to macroshock, microshock occurs with currents as low as 10μA.

The Skin Effect

The effect of electricity on a body structure is related to the magnitude and the frequency of the electrical current. As frequency increases in a conductor, the current tends to flow near the surface. This is known as the skin effect, if electrical current contacts a person. High frequency currents have a lower penetration through the skin. Low frequency currents have a higher penetration through the skin.

Electrical safety tests are scheduled on a regular basis for medical equipment in order to protect patients, staff and visitors in the hospital from being shocked. The scheduled maintenance, including electrical safety tests and operational tests, is known as preventive maintenance (PM). The accepted values for an electrical safety test are listed in Table 4.01.

Devices deemed nonmedical equipment by the manufacturer may exceed the recommended 500mA limit if reasonable grounding precautions are in place or isolation transformers can be implemented. This situation may occur with personal devices that patients, visitors, physicians, or staff members bring into the hospital.

ALL devices must be tested by the clinical engineering department for mechanical and electrical safety when entering a medical facility. Video cameras, radios, electric razors, electric hair dryers, laptop computers, and electronic video games commonly fall into this category.

Devices that are battery operated pose little or no threat to patient safety due to power isolation. Therefore, battery-operated power should be encouraged if personal electronic items are approved for use in the hospital. In addition to the electrical hazard, there is also a biocontamination hazard when personal items penetrate the skin or an open wound. Bacteria or viruses from the personal item may be transferred to the body of the patient, staff and/or visitors.

Table 4.01

NFPA Section 99 (1993 ed.) maximum allowable values for ground impedance and leakage current of medical devices

Maximum safe testing values for electronic connections of medical devices

Ground integrity	0.5 Ω
Wet Areas (hydrotherapy)	100 μA
General portable equipment	300 μA
Nonpatient care areas	500 μA

Table 4.02

Electric current values and associated physiological effects on the body

Body Response	Current in mA	Category of Current
Tingling or prickly feeling	1-5	Threshold
Physical pain	5-8	Pain Intensity
Muscles contract involuntarily [considered very dangerous since you can't let go of the object]	8-20	Let go
Muscles in the lungs become paralyzed – pain	>20	Paralysis
Uncontrollable contractions of the ventricles (large muscles) of the heart	80-1000	Fibrillation
Heart ventricles remain contracted, external burns, shock, death	1000-10,000	Defibrillation

Monitoring and Testing Devices

Ground Fault Current Interrupters

A *ground fault current interrupter* (GFCI) is the most common safety device found in hospitals. The National Electrical Code (NEC) also requires GFCIs in residential (home) hazardous areas. All wet areas of the hospital require GFCI receptacles.

A typical wet area in a hospital would be a hydrotherapy room or patient shower. A GFCI prevents the possibility of electric shock if both the ground and hot leads come in contact with the body simultaneously. Refer to the Figure 4.04 of a ground fault current interrupter.

If there is a difference of approximately 6mA for at least 0.2 seconds between the hot lead and the neutral lead, the sensing amplifier (differential amplifier) will cause both the hot and neutral contacts to open, shunting all electric current to the ground circuit. The sensing circuit utilizes an equal number of wire turns of the hot and neutral wires in opposite directions around a magnetic core (torroid). In the normal state, the inputs to the differential amplifier are equal, and therefore, the ideal output is zero (current in = current out). The creation of another circuit path in either the hot wire (input) or neutral wire (output) causes a current imbalance at the differential amplifier (Kirchhoff's Current Law), which results in an output of electric voltage from the differential amplifier to the solenoid relay, opening the contacts.

Figure 4.04

Diagram of a ground fault current interrupter (GFCI)

The two coils around the torroid are wrapped in opposite directions from the hot and neutral wires. Without loading, the corresponding output is zero volts. If either side of the coil has an increase or decrease in current due to loading, then the relay will be magnetically energized, shunting the output current to ground.

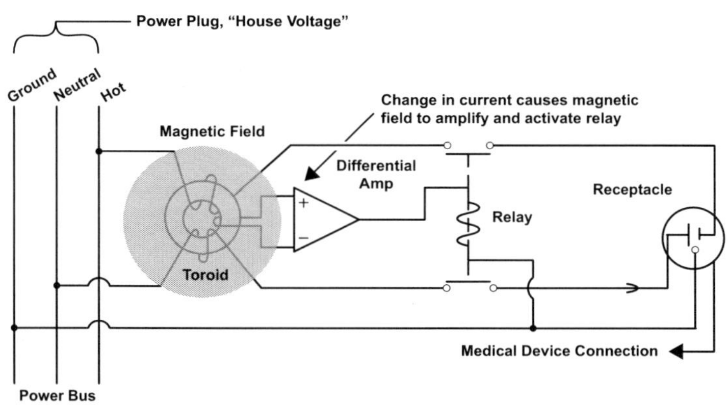

GFCIs are never used in an operating room setting. If current flow is interrupted to a surgical device during a procedure, there may be serious consequences or even death. If there is a problem with the circuit breaker or a medical device in a wet area of the surgical suite, it will be attended to immediately following the completed surgical procedure.

Figure 4.05 **GFCI wall outlet and inner circuit**

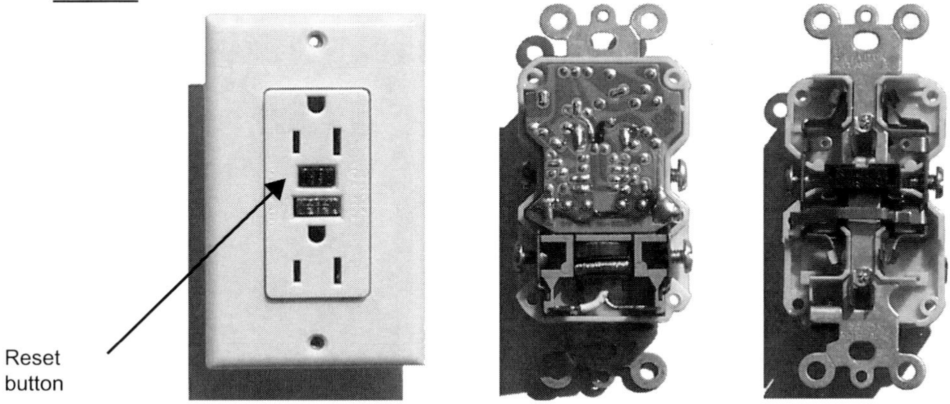

Line Isolation Monitors

Line isolation monitors (LIMs) are normally found in critical areas, such as the operating room of most hospitals. The purpose of the LIM is to monitor differences between the impedance in the hot and neutral leads of a particular device or room circuit. This is accomplished by measuring the difference in impedance between the hot lead through an ammeter to ground and current flowing from the neutral lead through an ammeter to ground. If this difference exceeds a certain limit, normally 2-5mA of current, an alarm is sounded. A LIM will not shunt current away from the circuit, as in the case of a GFCI. An alarm does not necessarily mean that the system must be shut down. In critical cases, power can remain on to allow surgical procedures to be completed.

Figure 4.06 **Diagram of a line isolation monitor**

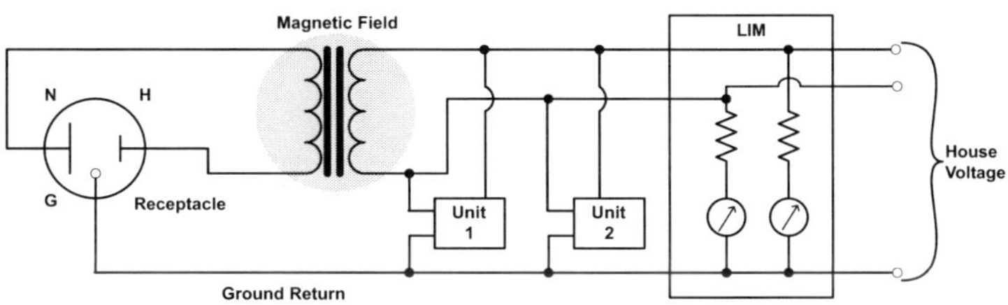

Line isolation monitor connected to medical devices (Unit 1 & Unit 2) commonly found in operating room settings for surgery and obstetrical operating suites.

Figure 4.07 **Line isolation monitor with visible coil**

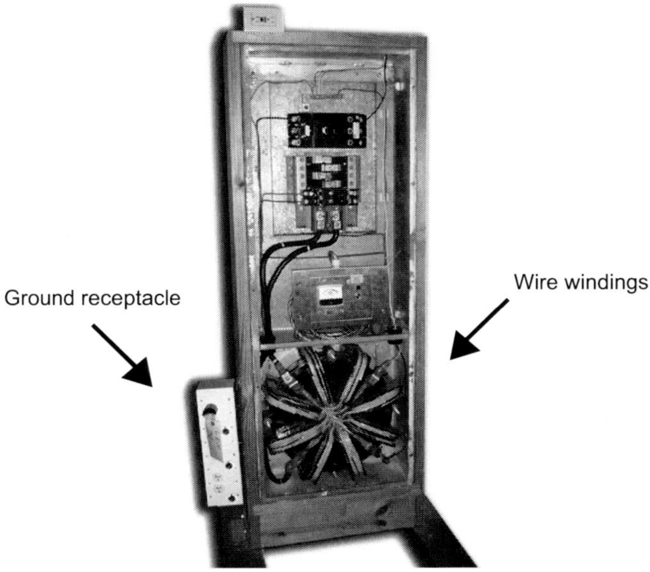

Isolation of power sources to prevent the hazard of electrical shock is an important consideration in the design of medical devices. Note that the wire windings on the equipment side of the isolation transformer are grounded to the ground receptacle of the power plug.

Electrical Safety Analyzer

Electrical safety analyzers are used as part of an ongoing preventive maintenance (PM) program and also to test devices entering a healthcare facility. The basic safety tests performed are 1) ground integrity (impedance from ground pin to chassis) and 2) leakage current (the unintentional flow of current from the chassis to the ground pin). This current may be due to mechanical disruptions or capacitive inductance. (Refer to NFPA 99 standards in Table 4.01.)

The device to be tested is plugged into the safety analyzer receptacle. All current entering the device being tested must first pass through the safety analyzer.

Leakage current is obtained with an open ground and either open hot or open neutral (forward and reverse current flow occurs in either position). Ground integrity is obtained by placing one lead test probe on the chassis or ground pin, with both neutral and hot leads open. In the calibration (Cal) position a normal reading should be 1mA.

Figure 4.08 Block diagram of medical device in position to perform electrical safety test

Note: Safety analyzer is positioned between wall outlet and the device to be tested.

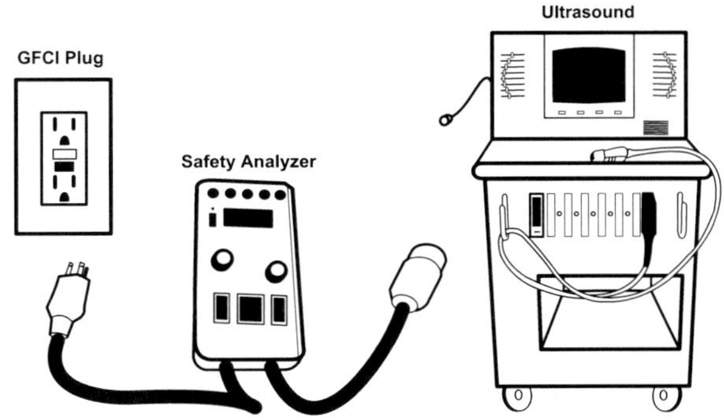

Figure 4.09 Safety analyzer

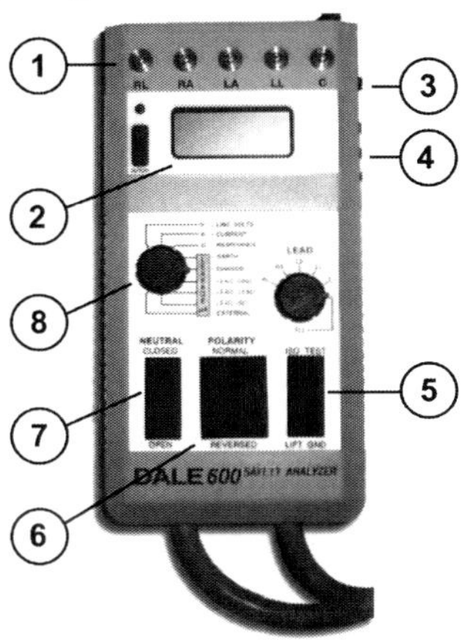

1. **ECG CONNECTORS:** Snap-on connectors to ECG leads.
2. **DISPLAY:** Shows result of the selected test measurement.
3. **LOAD SELECTOR SWITCH:** Selects the AAMI or the IEC 601-1 test load.
4. **TEST JACKS:** Calibrated outputs for resistance (1 Ohm) and leakage current (200 µA).
5. **GROUND SWITCH:** Temporarily opens the ground connection from device to analyzer.
6. **POLARITY SWITCH:** Selects Normal and Reverse polarity of the test receptacle and turns power off.
7. **NEUTRAL SWITCH:** Temporarily opens the neutral line from device to analyzer.
8. **SELECTOR SWITCH:** Selects desired test mode.

The Concept of Grounding

Normally, medical devices will be plugged into house voltage, and therefore, a brief review of electrical wiring and outlets is in order. All plugs used for medical devices must be heavy-duty, designed for extreme conditions and labeled (or equivalent to) hospital grade.

Hospital grade specifications are referenced in the National Electrical Code (NEC), American National Standards Institute (ANSI) section C73, and the National Fire Protection Association (NFPA) 70, section 410. The notation for hospital-grade power plugs is a green dot near the outside center of the hub. All hospital-grade power plugs must be the three-pronged variety. Most commercial electronic devices are equipped with two-prong plugs. This can present some safety concerns if these devices are brought into hospitals.

Three-Prong Plugs

Refer to the diagram of the three-pronged plug in Figure 4.10. The three wires connected to the three metal prongs are known as hot (H), neutral (N) and ground (G).

The *hot wire* is colored black for North American manufactured devices and brown for European and Japanese manufactured devices. It is called hot to describe it visually as delivering current flow into the device (conventional or Franklin current flow reference).

The *neutral wire* is colored white for North American manufactured devices and blue for devices manufactured in Europe and Japan. This wire is called neutral to describe visually an acceptance of current flow from the device (conventional or Franklin current flow reference). The hot and neutral wires are connected to the flat-spade prongs. The third wire (ground) is connected to the oval mid-line prong. North American made devices have solid green colored ground wires. European and Japanese manufactured devices have green with a yellow spiral stripe(s) to denote the ground wire. At the outlet, the hot wire will run through the conduit from the main power source for the facility. The neutral and ground wires run as parallel circuits, with the neutral wire acting as the return circuit for the power source and the ground wire attaching to the conduit that has an eventual connection to a metal stake in the earth, hence, the term *ground wire*. If the neutral wire becomes broken, current will flow to the ground wire. Lowered resistance increases the current through the hot wire, which is always connected to a fuse. When the current limit of the fuse is exceeded, the fuse element will open, causing the device to shut down. If the ground wire isn't available on the device, anyone touching the outer shell (chassis) or any conductive area would act as the ground wire in the absence of a neutral wire path, and the current would flow through the body. Ground wires also carry current away from the chassis if the hot wire breaks and touches the chassis.

Figure 4.10 **Hospital-grade power plug and corresponding wall outlet**

Hospital-grade plugs are certified by Underwriters Laboratories and require stringent physical specifications and testing.

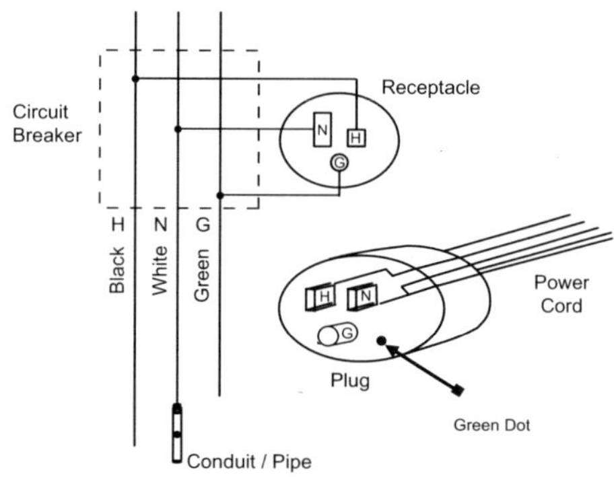

A green dot on the outer ring of the plug indicates that the plug is of hospital-grade quality. Hospital-grade quality electrical materials require more rigorous testing than those of consumer devices and are rated as Underwriters Lab (UL) quality.

Glossary of Terms

Electric shock: an electrical shock is an unwanted or unnecessary physiological response to current.

Ground fault current interrupters (GFCIs): the most common safety device found in hospitals that prevent the possibility of electric shock if both the ground and hot leads come in contact with the body simultaneously. All wet areas of the hospital require GFCI receptacles. (A typical wet area in a hospital would be a hydrotherapy room or patient shower.)

Ground wire: neutral and ground wires run as parallel circuits, with the neutral wire acting as the return circuit for the power source and the ground wire attaching to the chassis.

Hot wire: called hot to describe it visually as delivering current flow into the device (conventional or Franklin current flow reference).

Line isolation monitors: LIMs are normally found in critical areas such as the operating room of most hospitals. The purpose of the LIM is to monitor differences between the currents in the hot and neutral leads of a particular device or room circuit.

Macroshock: a physiological response to a current applied to the surface of the body that produces unwanted or unnecessary stimulation, muscle contractions or tissue damage.

Microshock: a physiological response to current applied to the surface of the heart that results in unwanted or unnecessary stimulation, muscle contractions or tissue damage. In contrast to macroshock, microshock occurs with currents as low as 10mA.

Neutral wire: called neutral to describe visually an acceptance of current flow from the device (conventional or Franklin current flow reference). The neutral and ground wires run as parallel circuits, with the neutral wire acting as the return circuit for the power source, and the ground wire attaching to the conduit that has an eventual connection to a metal stake in the earth, hence, the term ground wire.

One-hand rule: when inserting tools or touching any tool make sure only the holding hand has a possibility of contact with electric current. This prevents the creation of a completed circuit across the chest and heart, and returning through the chassis (conductive case) of the device.

Safety analyzers: a test device used as part of an ongoing preventive maintenance (PM) program and also to test devices entering a healthcare facility. The basic safety tests performed are 1) ground integrity (impedance from ground pin to chassis) and 2) leakage current (the unintentional flow of current from the chassis to the ground pin).

Voltage potentials: created when the voltage at one point is higher than a voltage at another point, with respect to the reference point or ground.

Chapter 4 Review Questions

Name:____

Date:____

1. Explain the difference between microshock and macroshock.

2. How does the one-hand rule provide protection from macro and microshock?

3. Explain the principle of operation of a ground fault current interrupter (GCFI).

4. Where would you expect to find GFCIs in the hospital setting?

5. Explain the principle of operation of a line isolation monitor (LIM).

6. Where would you expect to find LIMs in the hospital setting?

7. What is the purpose of a safety analyzer?

8. Draw a power cord used for a medical device and identify the hot, neutral and ground wires and corresponding plug pins.

9. What does the term "ground" or "grounding" mean?

Chapter 5: Medical Device Safety

After reading this chapter you will have an understanding and applied knowledge of:

- *The definition of preventive maintenance*
- *The definition of corrective maintenance*
- *The definition of calibration*
- *The relationship of device type versus inspection intervals*

Throughout the testing intervals for medical devices, there are three main types of maintenance that may be performed. These types of procedures may be scheduled or unscheduled, depending on the equipment or incident that occurs.

Preventive Maintenance

Preventive maintenance (PM) is defined as performing any nonfunctional repairs, cleaning, component replacement and any general maintenance in order to prevent improper and/or inadequate operation of a device. This is a scheduled maintenance procedure. In conjunction with preventive maintenance, electrical safety inspections may also be required. This type of maintenance can reduce possible electrical hazards and uncover any signs of possible failure in the future. These procedures include specific testing and standards that have been adopted by the facility using numerous federal and state regulations. Along with testing and performing preventive maintenance on a piece of equipment, there is an inspection sticker attached to the medical device to denote the type of inspection and possibly the next scheduled due date for the device. Within the PM procedure, there is a documentation trail (paper or paperless) that can be searched, if required, by any accrediting body, such as the JCAHO, during their unannounced inspection. Manufacturers may assign a PM maintenance schedule and print it in the device service manual. Your facility may use an alternate PM schedule (more frequent or less frequent) if you have documentation to support your decision. Any change in PM schedules from a standard interval must be approved by the hospital safety committee.

Corrective Maintenance

Corrective maintenance (CM), on the other hand, deals with the replacement of damaged or defective parts. Also included in this process is the possible partial or total calibration of a device. Corrective maintenance can occur during a PM if there is a specific part or area that is damaged and is not scheduled to be replaced during normal maintenance. An example of a part that is replaced during a PM would be something such as an oxygen sensor/cell. The normal steps for corrective maintenance entail receiving documentation or a phone call from a specific department and consequently repairing the device. As with PMs there is a work order or paper trail that is required. This documentation is essential to assist in determining possible trends of failure in different types of devices. This is also extremely helpful to technicians to assist them when referencing previous types of failures.

Calibration

Calibration of a device is defined as an adjustment or verification of a device's performance against a standard that is traceable back to the National Institute of Standards and Technology (NIST). This type of procedure may or may not be required during a PM or a CM, depending on the type of equipment or type of repair that is being performed. As with PMs and CMs, documentation is required for this process. There may also be a sticker applied to the device to denote the last calibration of the device.

Inspection Intervals

During normal operation of a healthcare facility, there are multiple types of computer programs utilized. Most facilities today use many different types of programs to manage and document their medical devices. Within these systems there are different intervals set for specific devices.

The intervals are usually determined by three or more areas: risk to patient, area of use and maintenance required. These three areas are usually given a numerical rating of 1-5. As each device is acquired, a staff individual will assign the unit a specific rating in each area. When this is done, there is a total number assigned. This number is sometimes called the *risk factor or equipment management number.* This number is put into a program, and dependent on the preset values assigned, a maintenance interval is set.

An example of this is an anesthesia unit. The area of use would be surgery; the risk to the patient is extremely high, and the maintenance required is above normal. With these three numbers calculated, this unit would have a maintenance interval of semi-annually or higher depending on the facility's policies and procedures. On the other hand, an exam lamp would be utilized in a clinical or exam area and would not pose a high risk to the patient and has little or no maintenance. This device would have a very low risk-factor number and be inspected on an annual basis.

Glossary of Terms

Corrective maintenance: the replacement of damaged or defective parts. Also included in this process is the possible partial or total calibration of a device.

Calibration: an adjustment or verification of a devices performance against a standard that is traceable back to the National Institute of Standards and Technology (NIST).

Inspection intervals: different testing intervals that are set for specific devices. The intervals are usually determined by three or more areas:

1) Risk to patient

2) Area of use

3) Maintenance required

Preventive maintenance: performing any nonfunctional repairs, cleaning, component replacement, and any general maintenance in order to prevent improper and/or inadequate operation of a device.

"Risk factor" or "equipment management number": a number dependent on the preset values assigned, a maintenance interval is set.

Chapter 5 Review Questions

Name____________________________________

Date_____________________________________

1) Explain the difference between corrective maintenance and preventive maintenance.

2) When might corrective maintenance and preventive maintenance be a part of the same procedure?

3) Explain how the "risk factor" is determined for medical devices.

4) Why must all PM and CM procedures be documented?

5) When might you change a PM interval from the standard inspection time interval?

6) Why would the biomedical repair shop make a decision to change the inspection time interval?

7) Which device would have a high risk factor and why?

a. Heart-lung machine

b. Defibrillator

c. Infusion pump

d. Wheelchair

Chapter 6: Fire Safety

After reading this chapter you will have an understanding and applied knowledge of:

- *The three components that are necessary for any fire*
- *The three types of fires and the extinguishing agents used for each*
- *The proper use and operation of a fire extinguisher*
- *The different types of fires associated with medical facilities*
- *The possible responsibilities of a BMET in a fire*
- *The RACE system most commonly used in healthcare facilities*

Fire safety is one of the most overlooked areas in most facilities. There are many different areas of fire safety that need to be followed to ensure a safe working environment. Throughout this chapter you will learn the different types of fires, the extinguishing agents for them and the responsibilities you may have as an employee within a medical facility.

The Fire Triangle

Fire itself is made up of three main parts. *The fire triangle,* as it is commonly called, consists of the following: fuel, oxygen and heat. All fires contain these elements and by removing any one of the three you can put out a fire.

Figure 6.01

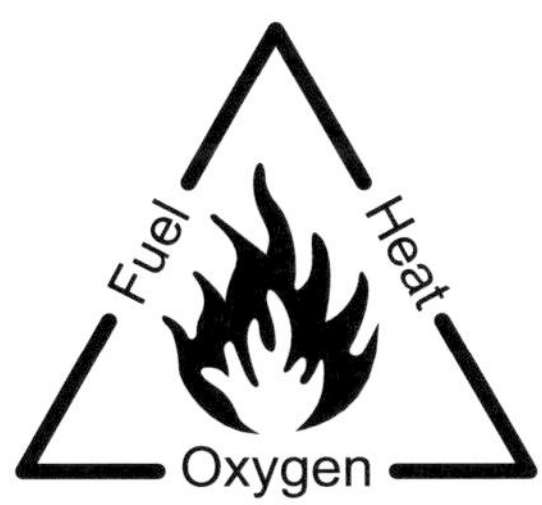

Types of Fires and Extinguishers

There are three main types of fires associated with healthcare facilities.

Class A fires are all fires associated with wood, paper or linens. The extinguishing agent to put out these fires is normally water. The extinguisher container for Class A fires is normally silver or chrome and filled with water and an antifreeze agent to keep the contents from freezing. This type of extinguisher is only used on Class A fires.

Class B fires are all fires associated with fuels or liquids. The extinguishing agent to put out these fires is normally a dry chemical agent. The agent suppresses the fire, removing the oxygen, thus putting out the fire. This type of extinguisher is normally red and is labeled for the class of fire.

Class C fires are all fires associated with electrical fires. The extinguishing agent to put out these fires is normally carbon dioxide. This agent is used to remove the oxygen from the fire and suppress the fire. This type of extinguisher is normally bright orange and is used for Class C fires.

In most facilities there are Class ABC fire extinguishers. They are red and contain both dry chemical and carbon dioxide. This type of extinguisher can be used on all three types of fires, but should be used with caution if used in the surgical area. The concern with using a Class A or B extinguisher in the surgical area is the contamination factor if the antifreeze or dry chemical agent enters an open wound during a procedure. Most facilities only install Class C extinguishers in the surgical area along with a fire hose system. This reduces the chance for contamination during a fire.

Figure 6.02

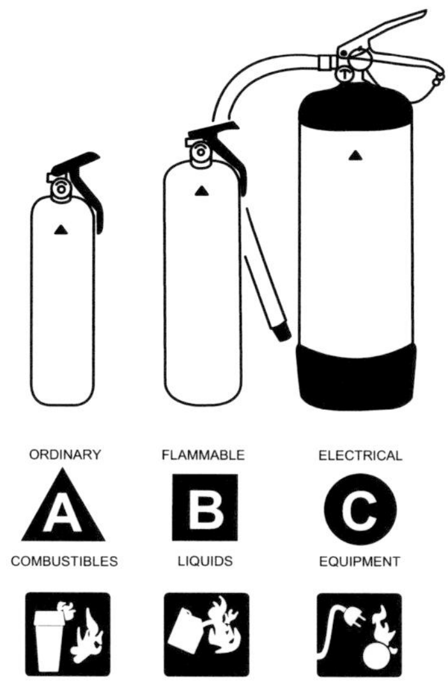

Using a Fire Extinguisher

If you ever need to use an extinguisher to put out a fire, you should know the proper technique. The *PASS* system should always be used. The PASS acronym stands for Pull the pin, Aim the hose at the base of the fire, Squeeze the trigger and Sweep the hose side to side. This technique will allow you to remove the oxygen from the base of the fire, eventually putting it out. All extinguishers are pressurized, therefore, you should be approximately 8-to-10 feet from the fire to reduce the chance of getting burned or causing your apparel to catch on fire. With these four steps, you can be successful in containing or suppressing a fire until the proper authorities have arrived.

Figure 6.03

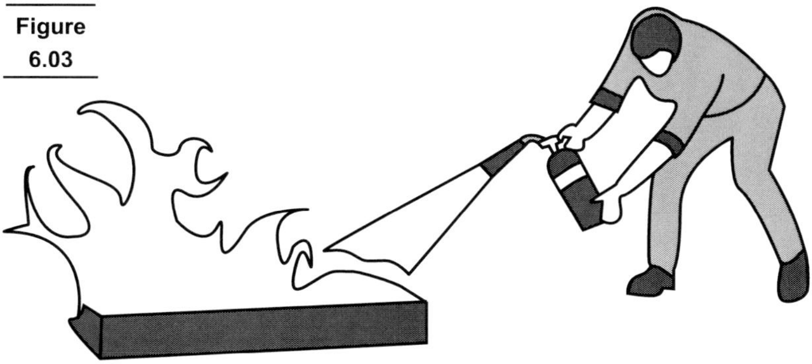

Fires in Medical Facilities

You may come across all three types of fires in medical facilities. Class A fires can be caused by fires from any type of paper product coming into contact with an open flame. They can also be caused by bed linens coming into contact with open flames or combustible materials. Class B fires, on the other hand, are caused by cooking oils or flammable liquids from spray cans coming into contact with open flames or heat sources. Class C fires are caused when excessive heat is produced by internal components within an electrical device. This is normally associated with aged equipment or equipment that is being used above its maximum capacity. All of these fires are life threatening and all precautions should be taken to keep them from happening.

As an employee within a medical facility, you may be asked to perform different tasks during a fire. The different tasks that you may be required to perform may include removing yourself from the building, fighting small fires, helping evacuate patients from the area of the fire, and cutting off medical gas supply valves. All of these tasks are necessary during a fire, and you will be notified of your specific duties during your orientation period at the facility.

RACE

If you come across a fire within a medical facility, you should use the *RACE* procedure. The RACE acronym stands for: Remove yourself from the area, Activate the alarm system by calling a specific number or pulling the fire alarm, Close all doors to help contain the fire to a specific area and Extinguish the fire or Evacuate the patients from the area.

Once again, as an employee of any medical facility, you may be asked to fulfill many different tasks during a fire. If you know the proper techniques, can distinguish the type of fire, and know the proper procedures, you can help reduce or eliminate the loss of life and property during a fire.

Glossary of Terms

Class A ***fires:*** fires associated with wood, paper or linen.

Class B ***fires:*** fires associated with fuels or liquids.

Class C ***fires:*** fires associated with electrical fires.

Class ABC fire extinguishers: most commonly used type of fire extinguisher in health care facilities. They are red and contain both dry chemical and carbon dioxide. This type of extinguisher can be used on all three types of fires.

Fire triangle: a fire warning label consisting of the following: fuel, oxygen and heat.

PASS: an acronym used to remember the procedures when using a fire extinguisher: Pull the pin, Aim the hose at the base of the fire, Squeeze the trigger, and Sweep the hose side to side.

RACE: an acronym used to remember the procedures used during a fire: Remove your self from the area, Activate the alarm system by calling a specific number or pulling the fire alarm, Close all doors to help contain the fire to a specific area, and Extinguish the fire or Evacuate the patients from the area.

Chapter 6 Review Questions

Name________________________________

Date_________________________________

1) What chemicals are contained in a Class A fire extinguisher?

2) When would you use a Class A fire extinguisher?

3) What chemicals are contained in a Class B fire extinguisher?

4) When would you use a Class B fire extinguisher?

5) What chemicals are contained in a Class C fire extinguisher?

6) When would you use a Class C fire extinguisher?

7) What chemicals are contained in a Class ABC fire extinguisher?

8) When would you use a Class ABC fire extinguisher?

9) As a healthcare professional, what are your responsibilities during a hospital fire?

Chapter 7: Natural and Community Disaster Precautions

After reading this chapter, you will have an understanding and applied knowledge of:

- *The definition of an internal disaster*
- *The definition of an external disaster*
- *The actions taken to protect patients and hospital staff during a natural or community disaster*
- *Examples of natural disasters*
- *The definition of a disaster plan*

Internal and External Disasters

The hospital serves as a community shelter and treatment center during a local disaster. Disasters are defined as events that cause great harm or injury. Disasters can occur within the facility itself (*internal disaster*) or outside the facility, affecting part, or all, of the local community (*external disaster*).

Natural disasters are considered external disasters. Examples of natural disasters are floods, earthquakes, hurricanes, tornados, mudslides, severe lightning storms, hail and ice storms, blizzards, and high winds. A natural disaster can be considered a community disaster due to the impact of a natural disaster on the healthcare response and resources.

A *community disaster* takes into consideration all forms of calamities that affect the community, both of natural and unnatural causes. Typical community disasters include multivehicle accidents, toxic gases, chemical or radioactive airborne hazards, and communications and electrical outages. Influenza and pandemic infections represent another community danger. Viruses that are spread in the air and infect the respiratory system represent the highest peril of all community disasters. Biohazard and other forms of terrorist threats are the unfortunate reality of external disasters that have evolved after the September 11, 2001, World Trade Center attacks. The healthcare response mechanism is the same in both natural and community disasters. The specific hazards involved will require specialized treatment areas.

Natural and community disasters present safety issues for those personnel who arrive at the scene of an impending disaster or its consequences. Local fire and police departments are usually the first to respond to a natural or community disaster. The fire and police departments provide information to the hospital about the number, type and severity of the injuries. The hospital is also notified by the National Weather Service in advance of a natural disaster, in order to provide time to notify the staff and call in additional staff if needed.

Disaster Plans

Each hospital or health center has a *disaster plan,* which contains detailed information pertaining to the type of disaster and emergency planning required. As an external disaster, natural and community disasters require a highly-coordinated communications network. The hospital must have accurate information from the scene of the disaster in order to communicate information "up-the-chain" to county public health centers and locally to other hospitals and emergency centers. Figure 7.01 illustrates a typical emergency communications network for disaster situations. The hospital communicates with all department directors in order to make special preparations for those injured in a natural or community disaster. The normal emergency room procedures are replaced with a *triage center*. The triage center directs patients brought to the hospital by emergency units to specialized areas, depending on the type and severity of their injuries.

The hospital clinical staff (nurses, physicians, clinical specialists) must divide their focus of care between those patients who have entered the hospital for personal medical procedures prior to the disaster and those patients who are entering the hospital due to their injuries from the disaster. Non-clinical staff, such as plant engineering and biomedical/clinical engineering, assist the clinical staff by assuming duties such as litter bearers and taking additional portable equipment to the triage areas.

The 2005 hurricane season demonstrated the need for a communications network that connected local communities, and state and federal agencies. The emergency effort must be coordinated to make the most efficient use of the resources available. There must also be a two-way communications network among those responding to the disaster and those providing outside relief for the disaster. Local community authorities have the most accurate information of local community members and special conditions that may arise in specific areas of the community. Communication of this local information is critical for a coordinated emergency response.

Figure 7.01

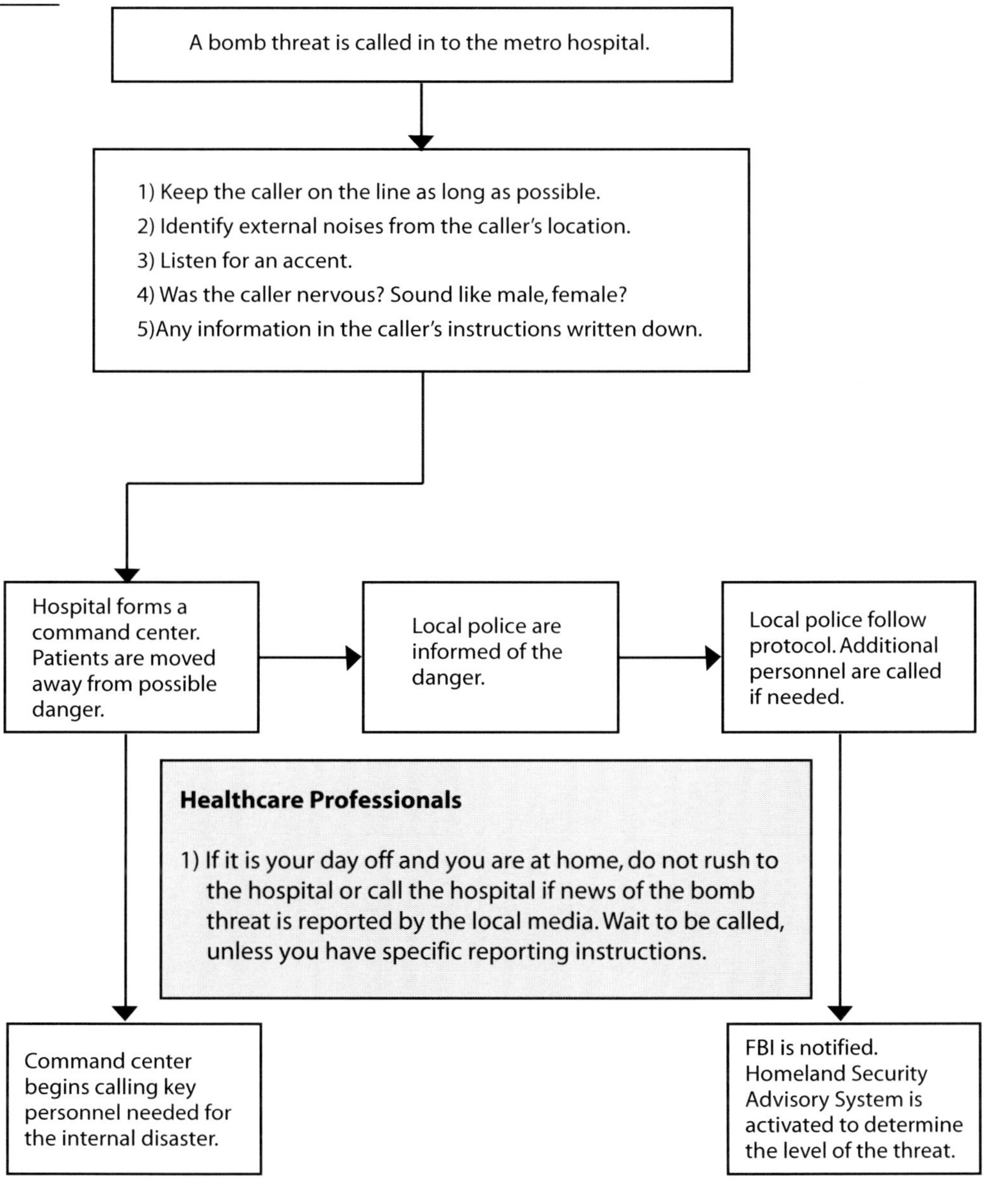
A bomb threat is called in to the metro hospital.
1) Keep the caller on the line as long as possible.
2) Identify external noises from the caller's location.
3) Listen for an accent.
4) Was the caller nervous? Sound like male, female?
5)Any information in the caller's instructions written down.
Hospital forms a command center. Patients are moved away from possible danger.
Local police are informed of the danger.
Local police follow protocol. Additional personnel are called if needed.
Healthcare Professionals
1) If it is your day off and you are at home, do not rush to the hospital or call the hospital if news of the bomb threat is reported by the local media. Wait to be called, unless you have specific reporting instructions.
Command center begins calling key personnel needed for the internal disaster.
FBI is notified. Homeland Security Advisory System is activated to determine the level of the threat.

Glossary of Terms

Community disaster: a disaster that takes into consideration all forms of calamities that affect the community both of natural and unnatural causes. Typical community disasters include multivehicle accidents, toxic gases, chemical or radioactive airborne hazards, and communications and electrical outages. Influenza and pandemic infections represent another community danger and are considered community disasters.

Disaster communications network: a two-way, infrastructure communications system that connects local communities, and state and federal agencies that is coordinated to make the most efficient use of the resources available.

Disaster plan: a preparation document that contains detailed information pertaining to the type of disaster and emergency planning required.

External disaster: disasters that occur outside the facility, affecting part or all of the local community.

Internal disaster: disasters that occur within the facility itself.

Natural disasters: disasters that occur from natural causes, such as floods, earthquakes, hurricanes, tornados, mudslides, severe lightning storms, hail and ice storms, blizzards, and high winds.

Triage center: a designated area (usually part of the emergency room) that directs patients brought to the hospital by emergency units, depending on the type and severity of their injuries.

Chapter 7 Review Questions

Name_______________________________

Date________________________________

1) What type of information should be included in a hospital disaster plan?

2) Why is a triage center necessary during a disaster?

3) Describe a community disaster that you personally experienced. Was the healthcare team effort coordinated?

Chapter 8: Internal Disaster Response and Planning

After reading this chapter, you will have an understanding and applied knowledge of:

- *Examples of internal disasters*
- *The actions taken to set up a command and communications center*
- *The role of the hospital or healthcare facility in an internal disaster*
- *The actions taken to protect and care for injured patients during an internal disaster*

Internal Disasters

Chapter 7 defined *internal disasters* as disasters that occur within the healthcare facility itself. Examples of internal disasters include fire, loss of water, broken water pipes or sewage pipes, loss of power, loss of internal communications systems, explosions, bomb threats and terrorist threats. Establishing the *command* and communications center is still the first priority of both internal and external disaster responses. Sending and receiving detailed and correct information is critical for an efficient and timely response to any emergency situation. Internal disasters are contained within the facility but may be due to an external source. Problem isolation is a critical second step or parallel process, along with the establishment of the communications center. Figure 8.01 illustrates a typical flow chart for internal disaster response.

Figure 8.01

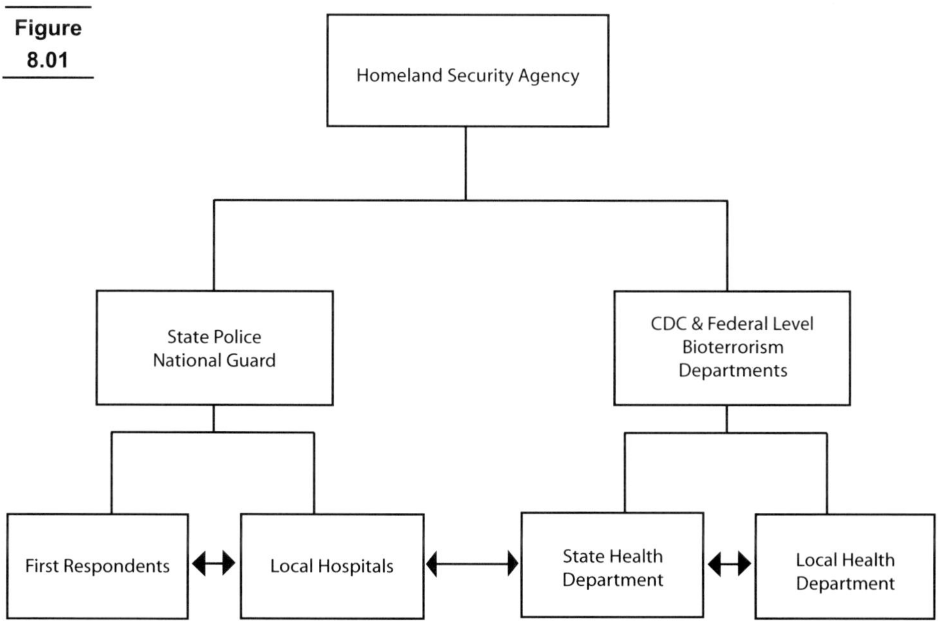

Command and Communications Center

The command and communications center is usually in close proximity to the emergency room. The command and communications center is essential for coordination of all resources. It should be set up and functional as quickly as possible. A preset area with limited communications equipment on standby provides the best method to rapidly place your communications system online.

The emergency room is the entry point for evaluation and treatment of all victims of a disaster. If internal communications are not functional, wireless communications must be implemented and coordinated. Cell phones are very useful in emergency situations, but strict call procedures must be observed. If a local or national news agency brings in their satellite links to broadcast information, local cell towers may be compromised and internal cell phone communication may become impossible.

A security perimeter must be maintained, and entry and exit of people responding to the disaster must be controlled. Name badges should be prepared as part of the emergency preparedness plan. Red clip-on badges that are labeled "staff nurse," "staff physician," "security," "staff maintenance," "medical equipment responder," etc., should be signed out at the command and communications center.

Family members and friends may overwhelm telephone land lines. Local television and radio stations should be part of the command and communications team. Local TV and radio stations can provide a number to call for information. This end-line communications network should be staffed with a bank of operators that provide information to the community. The operators should project calmness and the importance of the public staying away from the healthcare facility in order not to obstruct emergency traffic into and out of the healthcare facility.

Role of the Hospital or Healthcare Facility

The hospital's role is the same in both internal and external disasters. The hospital communicates with all department directors in order to reduce the hazards involved with an internal disaster and also to make special preparations for those who are injured or may become injured. The normal emergency room procedures are replaced with a triage center, which directs patients to specialized areas, depending on the type and severity of their injuries.

Establishment of interconnecting communications with law enforcement agencies and other health agencies is a key to the preparedness and response effort of the hospital and healthcare facility. Contingency plans for bomb threats, exposure to toxic gases and bioterrorism must be understood by all parties involved and readily executed when needed. Preparedness and the appropriate threat response are critical to the safety and containment efforts during an emergency. The best means of assuring preparedness is through planned exercises. If a problem is identified during an exercise, it can be corrected before it adds to the calamity of the actual disaster.

If you are a staff member at home during a disaster, you should understand your role. Unless you are a member of a critical care team, you should remain at home until you are contacted by your supervisor. Calling the hospital will only create further congestion of communications systems. Driving to the hospital may place you in the direct path of the disaster or interfere with emergency vehicle traffic.

Each member of the healthcare team will have a specific task detailed in the hospital *disaster preparedness plan*. An internal disaster will have a containment action, which is normally not part of the external disaster action plan. Establishment of the communications center is, however, always the first action taken during a disaster. Simultaneous actions will be occurring in other areas of the hospital. One group will be assigned to locate and evaluate the internal disaster. Another group will be assigned to remove patients and visitors from the dangers involved with the disaster. Coordination of these task groups will be the responsibility of the command and communications center.

Strategic areas of care will be set aside for injured patients, guests and staff. These strategic care areas will be established based on the information received from the assigned specialty groups evaluating their assigned areas. Some strategic care areas may be established as part of the disaster preparedness plan.

Glossary of Terms

Internal disasters: catastrophic events that include fire, loss of water, broken water pipes or sewage pipes, loss of power, loss of internal communications systems, explosions, bomb threats and terrorist threats within a health care facility.

Command and communications center: an area containing communications equipment that directs first responder units and for coordination of all resources during a disaster.

Disaster preparedness plan: a detailed document that provides action information for each department of the hospital during a disaster. Each member of the healthcare team will also have assignments, which are specific for the type of disaster and the qualifications of the team. Strategic areas of care will also be included in the plan, based on the type and severity of the injured patient.

Chapter 8 Review Questions

Name_______________________________

Date________________________________

1) Why are planned or mock disaster exercises important for disaster preparedness?

2) If you are a hospital employee at home and a tornado warning appears on your television, what actions should be taken?

3) Based on the knowledge of your particular healthcare career, what assignments should you expect during a disaster?

Chapter 9: Terrorist Response and Planning

After reading this chapter, you will have an understanding and applied knowledge of:

- *The role of the hospital or healthcare facility in an internal terrorist threat*
- *The role of the hospital or healthcare facility in an external terrorist threat*
- *The actions taken to set up a command and communications center during a terrorist threat*
- *Pathological agents associated with terrorist threats*

The World Trade Center bombing on February 26, 1993, the Oklahoma City bombing by a member of a Michigan militia organization on April 19, 1995, and the September 11, 2001, plane hijacking and ensuing destruction of the World Trade Center in New York City began a new era and a new paradigm for terrorist response and planning in the United States. A response effort for victims of terrorist activities must be well coordinated, in both healthcare and law enforcement activities. The communications system must be on a state and national level. Never before in the history of the United States have hospitals and healthcare facilities been tasked with such a preparedness endeavor.

Role of the Hospital or Healthcare Facility

As stated in Chapters 7 and 8, the role of the hospital or healthcare facility remains much the same in both internal and external disasters. The primary difference is the scope of the triage effort and the command and communications center network. The hospital will serve as a community shelter and treatment center during an external terrorist threat. If there is a terrorist threat within the hospital, the staff and local law enforcement members must isolate the threat and remove patients, visitors and staff from high risk areas. Triage areas may be set up within the hospital, or it may be necessary to have triage areas outside the hospital if there is a danger of biological, chemical or radiation exposure within the hospital.

The most critical factor in a terrorist threat is protecting the healthcare emergency responder staff from exposure to pathological agents. There must also be a stringent effort by the emergency responder staff to keep the threat isolated and not become a means of transporting the pathological agent into the triage areas. Mass causalities are generally associated with terrorist activities. If the medical personnel are exposed to the pathological agents, the ability to care for injured victims of terrorist activity is limited. *First responders* are members of the local disaster team that arrive at the scene of an emergency and provide both security activity and medical treatment and transport. Examples of first responders are firefighters, local police and emergency medical professionals.

The Homeland Security Act of 2002 was established in the aftermath of the September 11, 2001, terrorist attacks to coordinate the efforts of first responders nationwide. *The Department of Homeland Security* (DHS) was also put into operation by presidential executive order following what has become known as the 9-11 disaster. The Department of Homeland Security has a six-point agenda:

1) Increase overall preparedness

2) Create better transportation security systems to remove people and cargo more securely and efficiently

3) Strengthen border security and interior enforcement and reform immigration processes

4) Enhance information sharing with our partners

5) Improve DHS financial management, human resource development, procurement and information technology

6) Realign the DHS organization to maximize mission performance

In order to better prepare for terrorist threats and pandemics, the Centers for Disease Control and Prevention (CDC) established the *Coordinating Office for Terrorism Preparedness and Emergency Responses*, which provides a strategic plan for regional and local health centers to prepare them as first responders. The Centers for Public Health Preparedness program, which coordinates local and state mass causality and terrorist response, receives strategic planning from the CDC and is a responsibility of the Coordinating Office for Terrorism Preparedness and Emergency Responses.

The Actions Taken to Set Up a Command and Communications Center During a Terrorist Threat

The command and communications center of operations must follow standards in communications equipment used and activity established by the Centers for Public Health Preparedness program. The scale of communications coordination is on a national level and begins with first responders and state health departments at the local level. The CDC and the *U.S. Department of Health and Human Services* are the upper level of the command and communications center receiving directions from the Department of Homeland Security. The CDC monitors and evaluates mock training exercises to ensure there is an efficient flow of communications and resources from the local, city and state levels upward to the national level.

Pathological Agents

Bioterrorism is a recent form of terrorist threat for citizens of the United States. Biological warfare has been used in some form for centuries by several countries. The threat of exposing entire populations to deadly organisms and toxins is now a reality of the 21st century. Typical bioterrorism agents are classified in order of highest risk as Category A, B and C disease/agents by the CDC.

Category A agents include anthrax, botulism, plague, smallpox, tularemia, and viral hemorrhagic fevers such as Ebola. Agents in Category A can be easily disseminated or transmitted from one person to another, result in high mortality rates and have the potential for mass causalities, might cause public panic and social disruption, and require special action for public health preparedness.

Category B agents include brucellosis, epsilon toxin of clostridia perfringens, food threats such as e coli, salmonella and shigella, glanders, psittacosis, Q fever, ricin, staph enterotoxin B, typhus fever, viral encephalitis, and water threats. Agents in Category B are moderately easy to disseminate, result in moderate morbidity rates and low mortality rates, and require specific enhancements of CDC's diagnostic capacity and disease surveillance.

Category C agents include emerging pathogens that may be spread in large numbers to the general public.

Glossary of Terms

Category A bioterrorism agents: pathogens that have the highest risk of causing mass causalities. They include anthrax, botulism, plague, smallpox, tularemia, and viral hemorrhagic fevers such as Ebola. Agents in Category A can be easily disseminated or transmitted from one person to another, result in high mortality rates and have the potential for mass causalities, might cause public panic and social disruption, and require special action for public health preparedness.

Category B bioterrorism agents: pathogens that have a moderate risk of causing mass causalities. They include brucellosis, epsilon toxin of clostridia perfringens, food threats such as e coli, salmonella and shigella, glanders, psittacosis, Q fever, ricin, staph enterotoxin B, typhus fever, viral encephalitis, and water threats. Agents in Category B are moderately easy to disseminate, result in moderate morbidity rates and low mortality rates, and require specific enhancements of CDC's diagnostic capacity and disease surveillance.

Category C bioterrorism agents: emerging pathogens that may be spread in large numbers to the general public.

Coordinating Office for Terrorism Preparedness and Emergency Responses: a branch of the CDC that provides strategic planning and resources for state and local public health preparedness programs.

US Department of Health and Human Services: a national governmental agency that has jurisdiction over the Centers for Disease Control and Prevention.

The Department of Homeland Security: a national governmental agency established under the Homeland Security Act of 2002. This agency has broad powers to protect the United States against subversive acts.

First responders: members of the local disaster team that arrive at the scene of an emergency and provide both security activity and medical treatment and transport. Examples include firefighters, local police and emergency medical professionals.

The Homeland Security Act of 2002: established in the aftermath of the September 11, 2001, terrorist attacks to coordinate the efforts of first responders nationwide.

Chapter 9 Review Questions

Name____________________________________

Date_____________________________________

1) Explain the role of each of the following agencies or units in a mass causality disaster.

   a. first responders

   b. Department of Homeland Security

   c. US Department of Health and Human Services

   d. Centers for Disease Control and Prevention

   e. Coordinating Office for Terrorism Preparedness & Emergency Responses

2) How would your role as a healthcare professional change during a mass causality disaster compared to an internal disaster?

Appendix A: Safety Signs

Hazards vs PPE (minimum PPE requirements)

Hazard	Eyes	Face	Body/Hands
Any laboratory or general use of chemicals	Safety glasses (all times in lab)		Normal work/lab attire (no sandals, shorts, etc) with over-garment (smock, lab coat, or coveralls), & gloves
Use of corrosive chemicals, strong oxidizing agents, carcinogens, mutagens, etc.	Chemical splash goggles	Full face shield over goggles (if gallon or more liquid)	Resistant gloves (see glove selection guide), resistant apron or over-garment (full protective suit for work with over 5 gal corrosive liquids)
Sharp objects, glass, insertion of tubes into stoppers	Safety glasses		Heavy cloth barrier or leather gloves
Temperature extremes	Safety glasses (goggles if possible splash)	Recommend full face shield (large quantity gas/liquid or sparking)	Insulated gloves for ovens, furnaces, cryogenics & devices over 100C or below -1C, use over-garment for hot/cold liquids & sparking

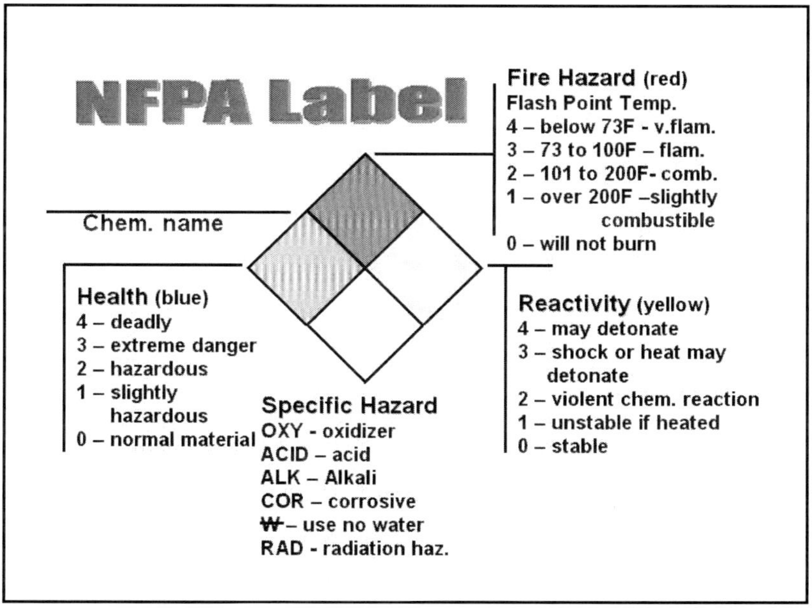

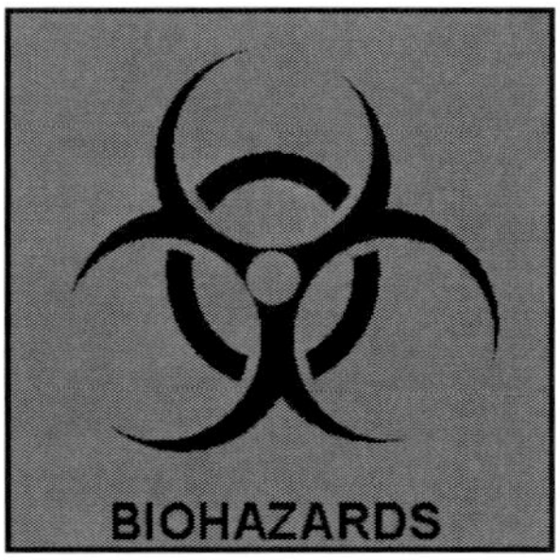
BIOHAZARDS

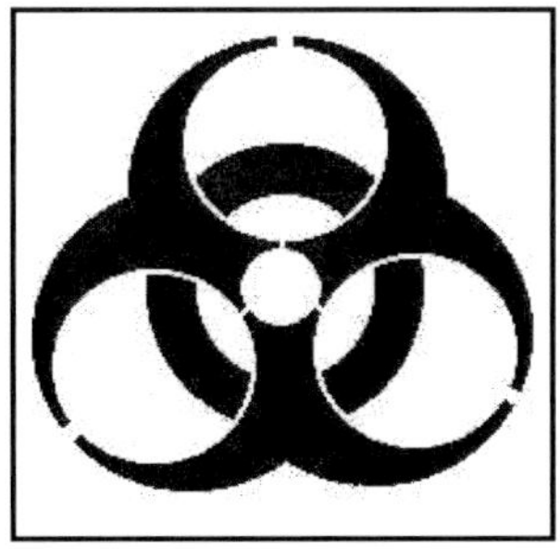

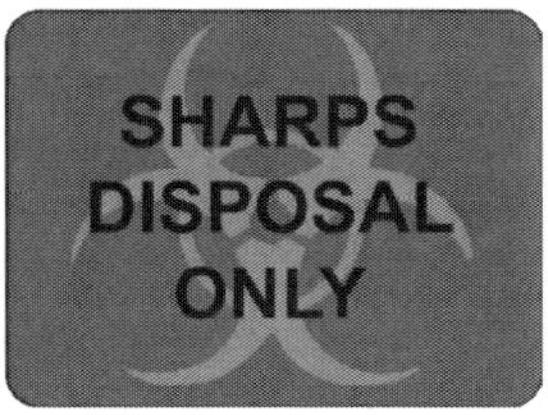
SHARPS
DISPOSAL
ONLY

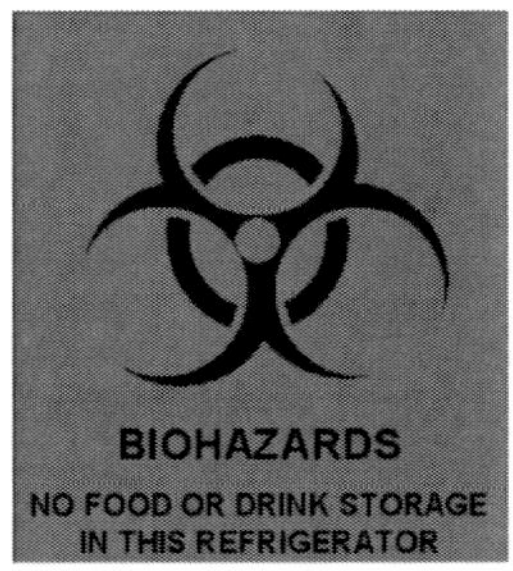
BIOHAZARDS
NO FOOD OR DRINK STORAGE
IN THIS REFRIGERATOR

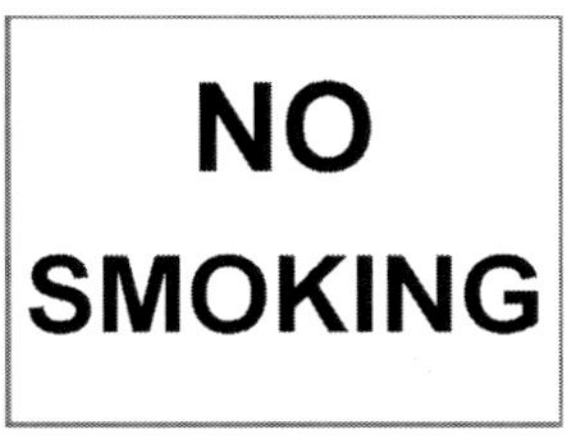
NO
SMOKING

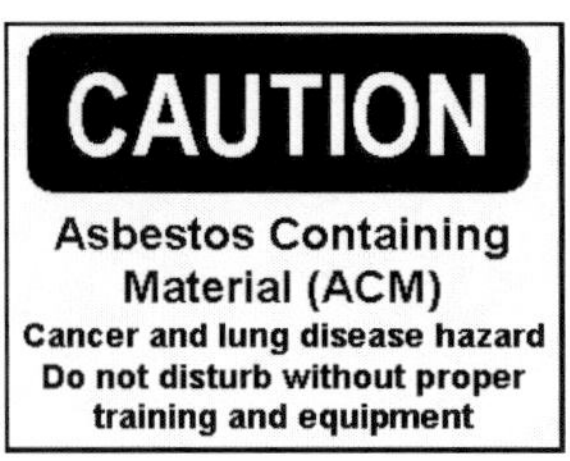
CAUTION
Asbestos Containing
Material (ACM)
Cancer and lung disease hazard
Do not disturb without proper
training and equipment

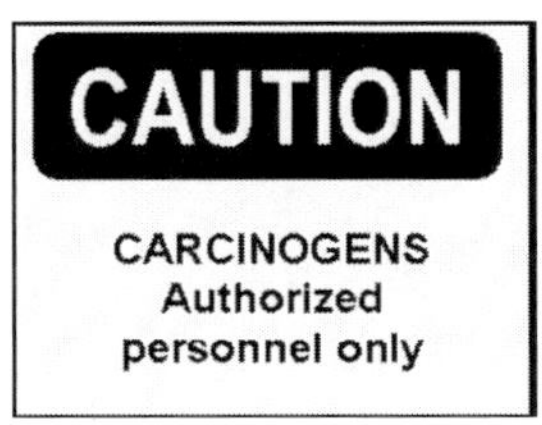
CAUTION
CARCINOGENS
Authorized
personnel only

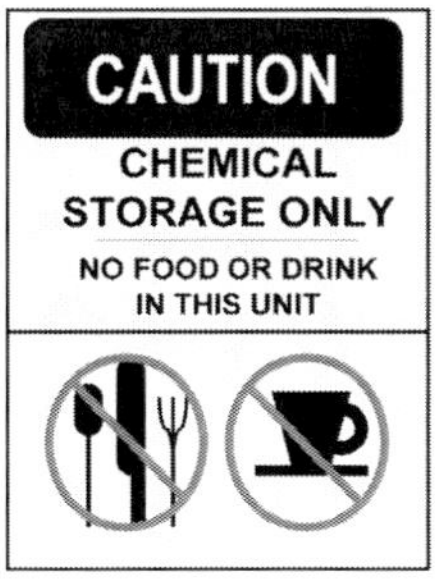
CAUTION
CHEMICAL
STORAGE ONLY
NO FOOD OR DRINK
IN THIS UNIT

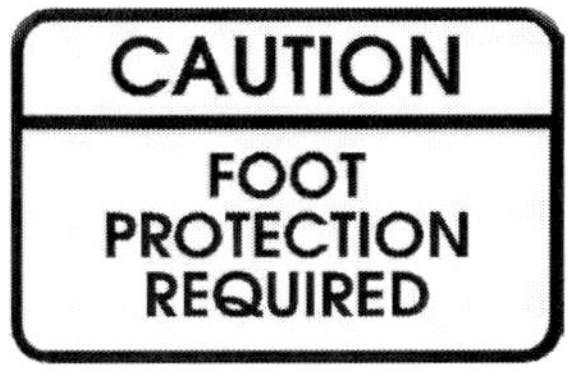
CAUTION
FOOT
PROTECTION
REQUIRED

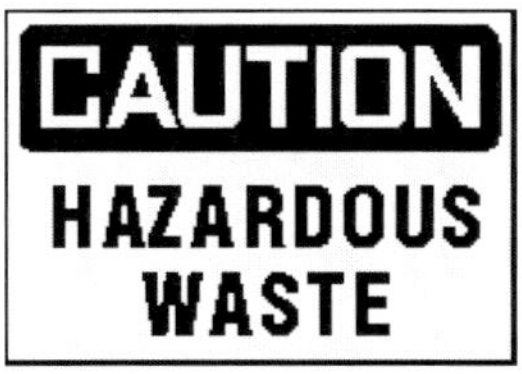
CAUTION
HAZARDOUS
WASTE

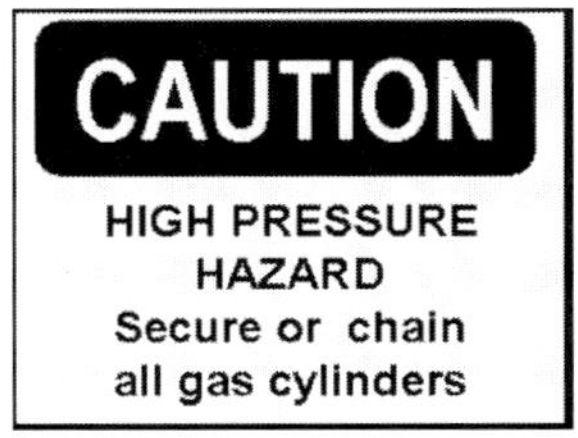
CAUTION
HIGH PRESSURE
HAZARD
Secure or chain
all gas cylinders

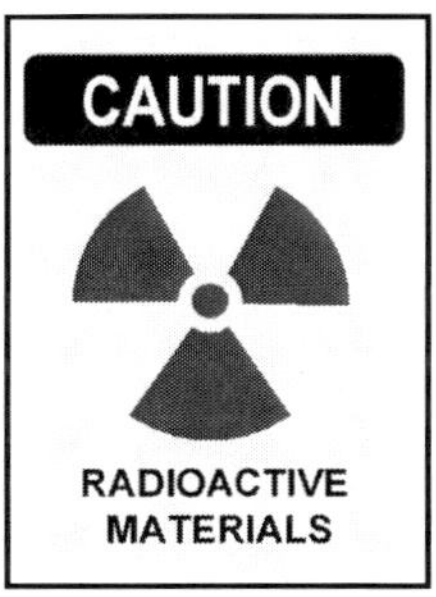
CAUTION
RADIOACTIVE
MATERIALS

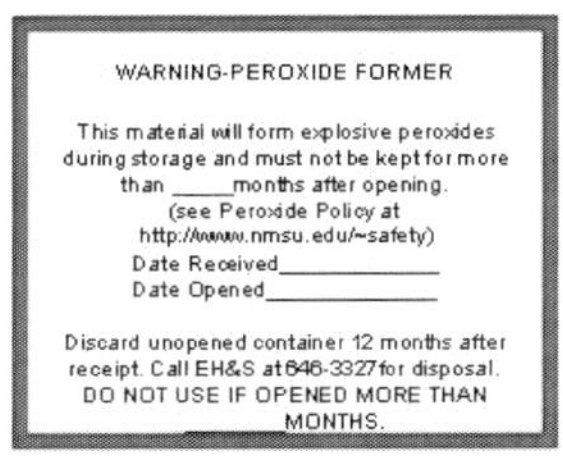
WARNING-PEROXIDE FORMER
This material will form explosive peroxides
during storage and must not be kept for more
than _____months after opening.
(see Peroxide Policy at
http://www.nmsu.edu/~safety)
Date Received_____________
Date Opened_______________
Discard unopened container 12 months after
receipt. Call EH&S at 646-3327 for disposal.
DO NOT USE IF OPENED MORE THAN
__________MONTHS.

BE SAFE
Always wash
hands to
remove residue
before leaving

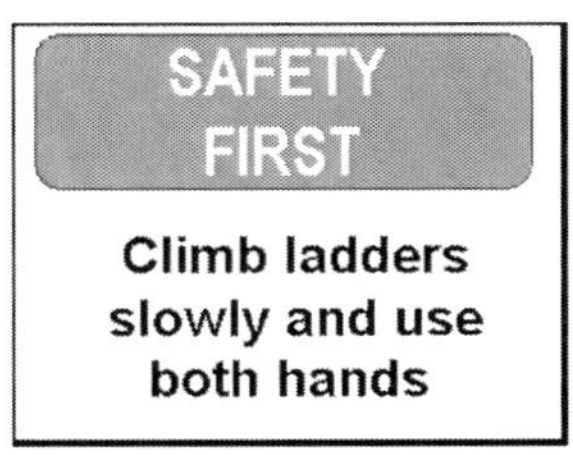
SAFETY
FIRST
Climb ladders
slowly and use
both hands

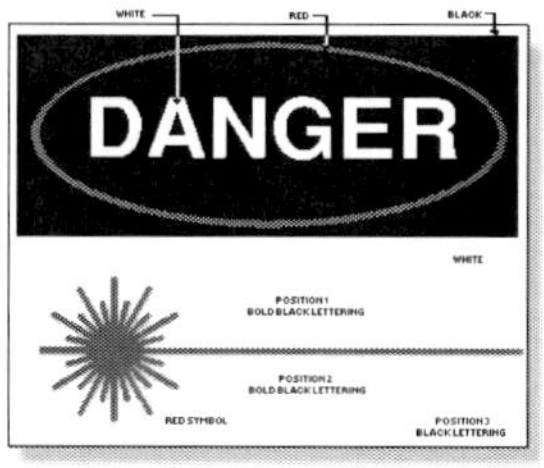
WHITE
RED
BLACK
DANGER
WHITE
POSITION 1
BOLD BLACK LETTERING
POSITION 2
BOLD BLACK LETTERING
RED SYMBOL
POSITION 3
BLACK LETTERING

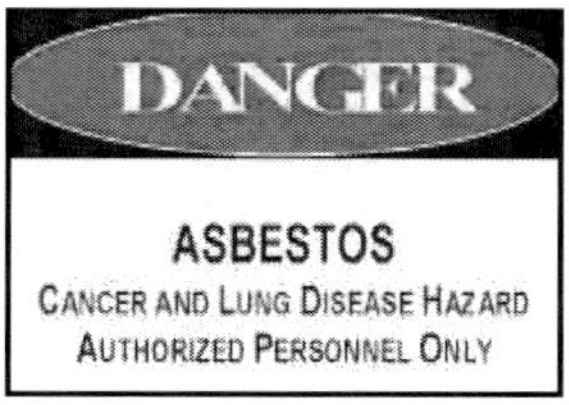
DANGER
ASBESTOS
CANCER AND LUNG DISEASE HAZARD
AUTHORIZED PERSONNEL ONLY

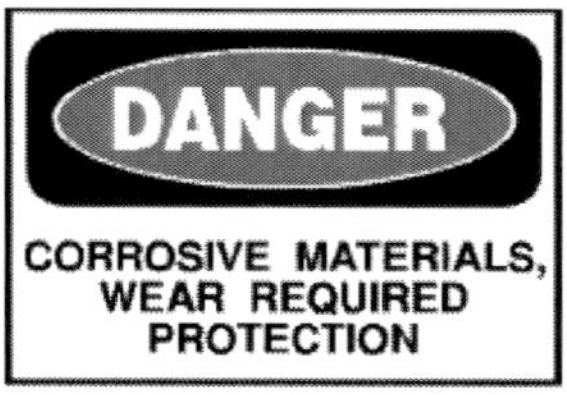
DANGER
CORROSIVE MATERIALS,
WEAR REQUIRED
PROTECTION

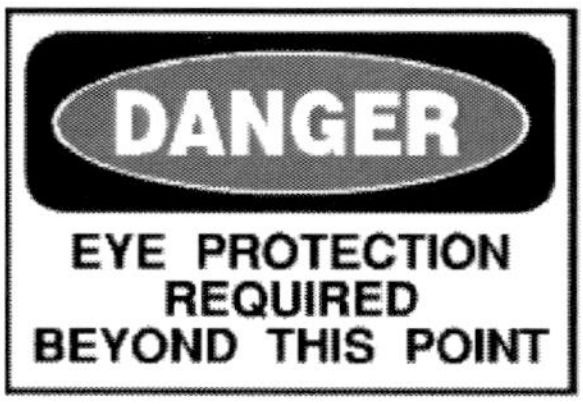
DANGER
EYE PROTECTION
REQUIRED
BEYOND THIS POINT

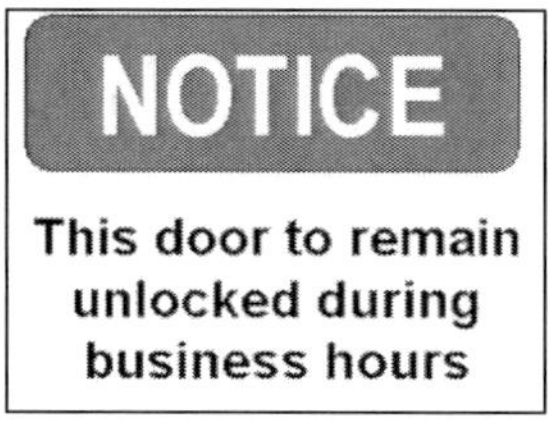
NOTICE
This door to remain
unlocked during
business hours

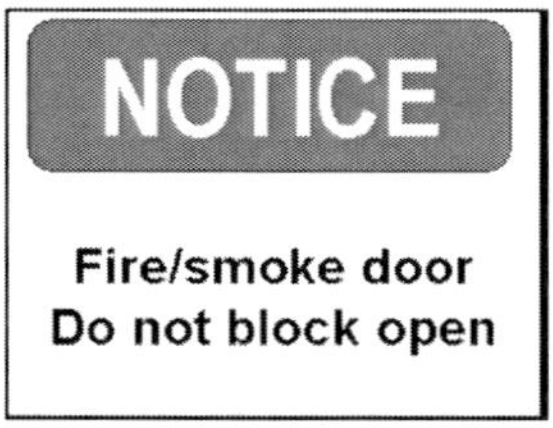
NOTICE
Fire/smoke door
Do not block open

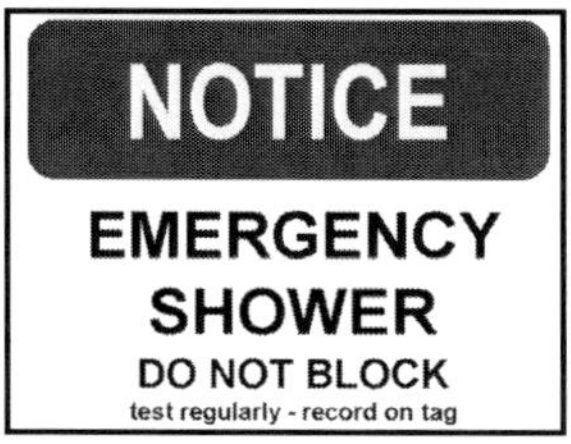
NOTICE
EMERGENCY
SHOWER
DO NOT BLOCK
test regularly - record on tag

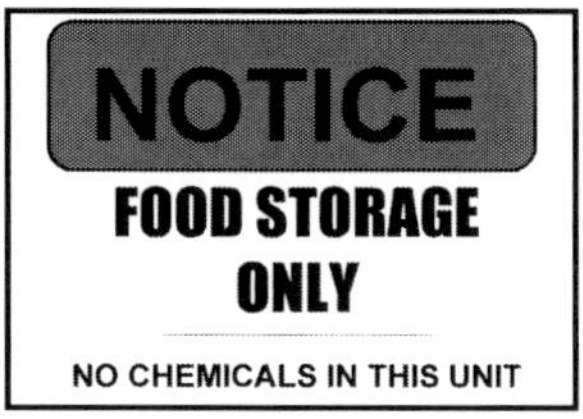
NOTICE
FOOD STORAGE
ONLY
NO CHEMICALS IN THIS UNIT

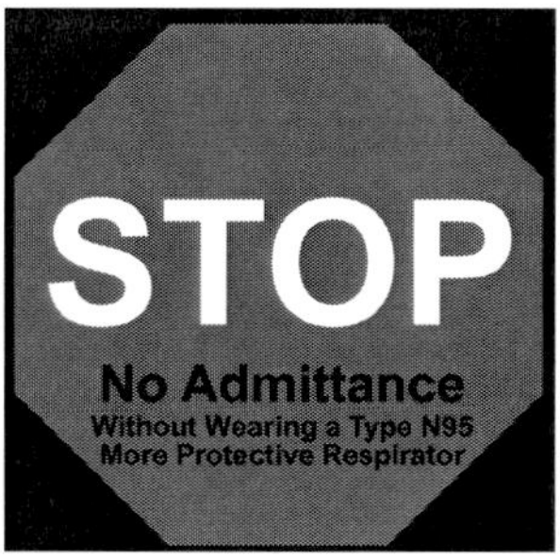
STOP
No Admittance
Without Wearing a Type N95
More Protective Respirator

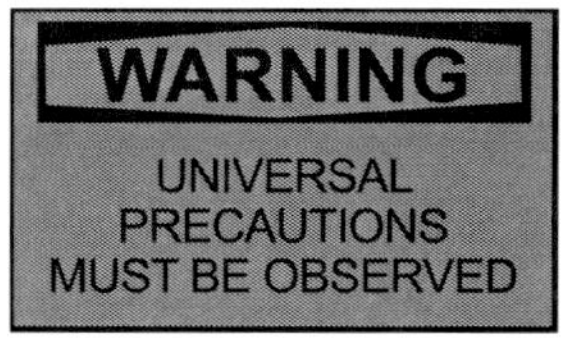
WARNING
UNIVERSAL
PRECAUTIONS
MUST BE OBSERVED

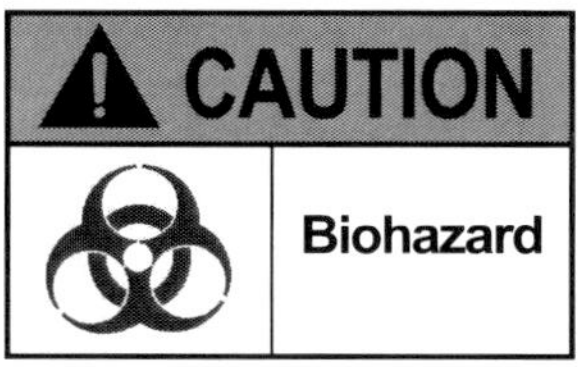
CAUTION
Biohazard

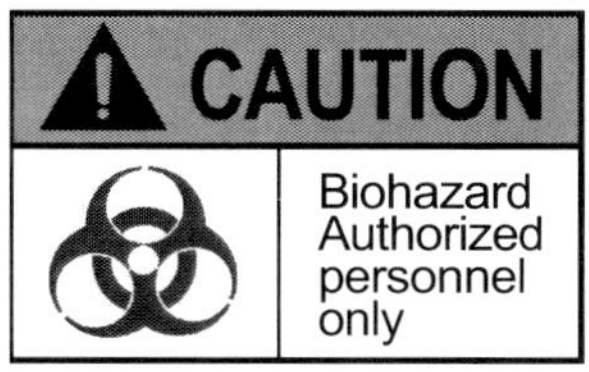
CAUTION
Biohazard
Authorized
personnel
only

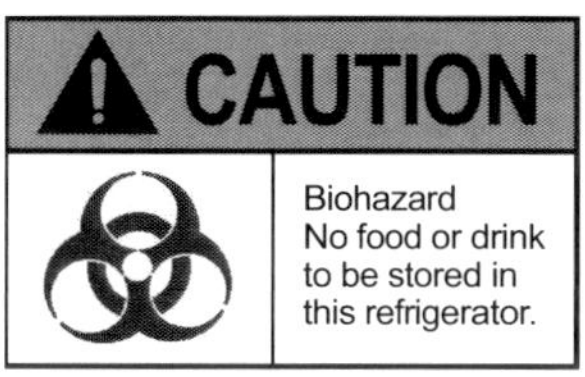
CAUTION
Biohazard
No food or drink
to be stored in
this refrigerator.

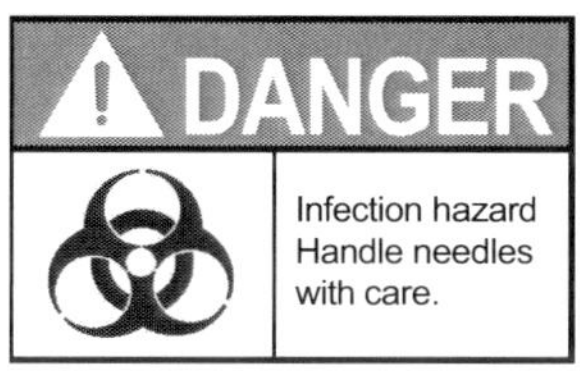
DANGER
Infection hazard
Handle needles
with care.

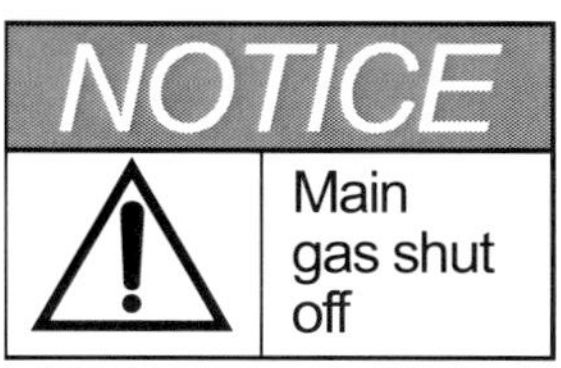
NOTICE
Main
gas shut
off

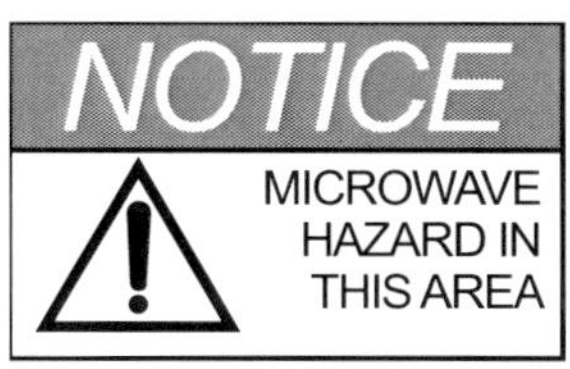
NOTICE
MICROWAVE
HAZARD IN
THIS AREA

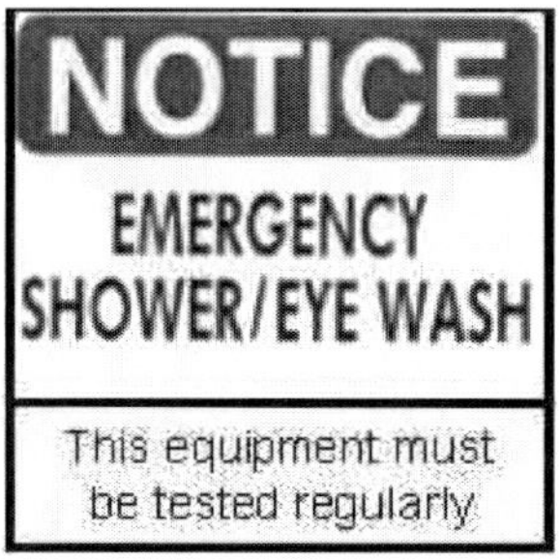
NOTICE
EMERGENCY
SHOWER/EYE WASH
This equipment must
be tested regularly

CORROSIVE
MATERIALS

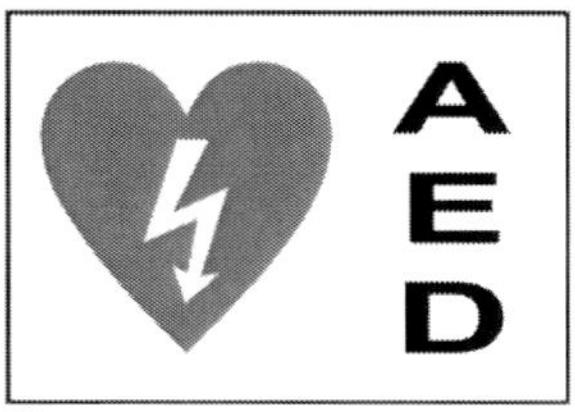
AED

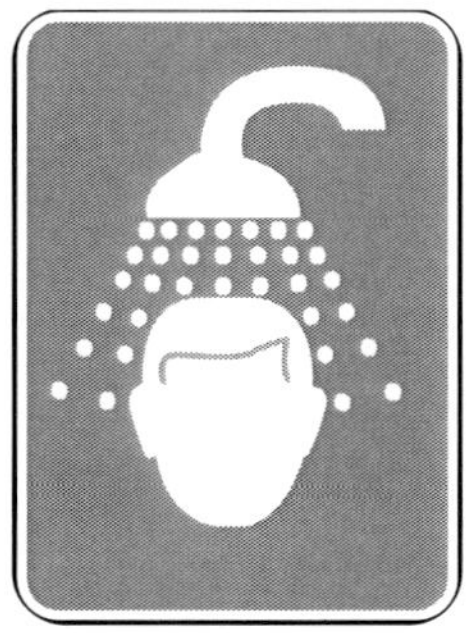

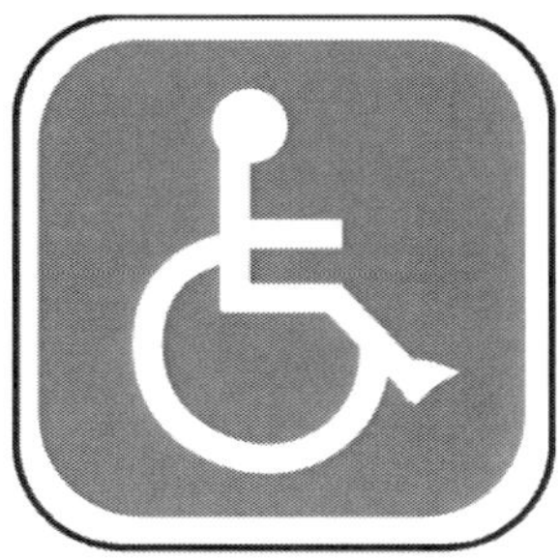

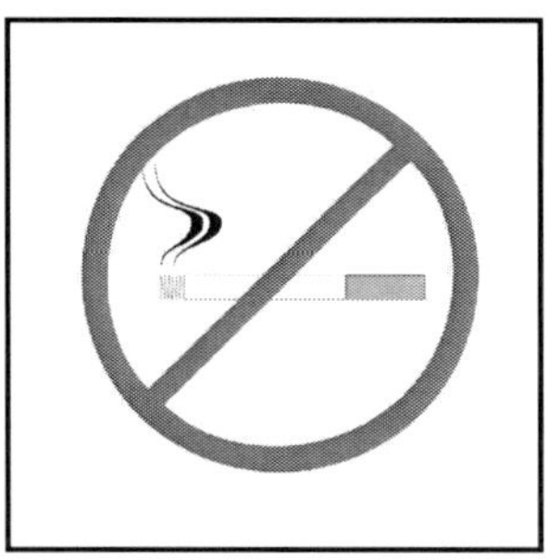

Appendix B: Useful Web Sites

AAMI
Association for the Advancement of Medical Instrumentation
www.aami.org

ANSI
American National Standards Institute
www.ansi.org

ASHE
American Society for Healthcare Engineering
www.ashe.org

ATSDR
Agency for Toxic Substances and Disease Registry
www.atsdr.cdc.gov/index.html

CCEHIP
Coordinating Center for Environmental Health and Injury Prevention
www.cdc.gov/about/organization/ccehip.htm

CoCHP
Coordinating Center for Health Promotion
http://www.cdc.gov/cochp/

CDC
Centers for Disease Control and Prevention
www.cdc.gov

CDRH
Center for Devices and Radiological Health
www.fda.gov/cdrh

COGH
Coordinating Office for Global Health
www.cdc.gov/nchstp/od/nchstp.html

DHHS
Department of Health and Human Services
www.hhs.gov

DHS
Department of Homeland Security
www.dhs.gov

ECRI
Emergency Care Research Institute
www.ecri.org

EPA
Environmental Protection Agency
www.epa.gov

FBI
Federal Bureau of Investigation
www.fbi.gov

FCC
Federal Communications Commission
www.fcc.gov

FDA
Food and Drug Administration
www.fda.gov

HIPPA
Health Insurance Portability and Accountability Act
www.hhs.gov/ocr/hipaa

ISO
International Organization for Standardization
www.iso.org

JCHA
The Joint Commission on Accreditation of Hospitals
www.jointcommission.org

MQSA
Mammography Quality Standards Act
www.fda.gov/cdrh/mammography/mqsa-rev.html

NCBDD
National Center on Birth Defects and Developmental Disabilities
http://www.cdc.gov/ncbddd

NCCDPHP
National Center for Chronic Disease Prevention and Health Promotion
www.cdc.gov/nccdphp

NCEH
National Center for Environmental Health
www.cdc.gov/nceh

NCHHSTP
National Center for HIV/AIDS, Viral Hepatitis, STD, and TB Prevention
www.cdc.gov/nchstp/od/nchstp.html

NCHM
National Center for Health Marketing
www.cdc.gov/healthmarketing

NCHS
National Center for Health Statistics
www.cdc.gov/nchs/

NCID
National Center for Infectious Diseases
www.cdc.gov/Ncidod

NCIPC
National Center for Injury Prevention and Control
www.cdc.gov/ncipc/ncipchm.htm

NCPHI
National Center for Public Health Informatics
www.cdc.gov/ncphi/

NFPA
National Fire Protection Association
www.nfpa.org

NIOSH
National Institute for Occupational Safety and Health
www.cdc.gov/niosh/

NIP
National Immunization Program
www.cdc.gov/Nip

NIST
National Institute of Standards and Technology
www.nist.gov

NOPHG
National Office of Public Health Genomics
www.cdc.gov/genomics

NRC
Nuclear Regulatory Commission
www.nrc.gov

NWS
National Weather Service
www.nws.noaa.gov

OSHA
Occupational Safety Health Administration
osha.gov

SMDA
Safe Medical Devices Act
www.fda.gov/cdrh/modact/smdatran.html

UL
Underwriters Laboratories
www.ul.com

WHO
World Health Organization
www.who.int/en

Index

V-W

About the Authors

Nicholas Cram

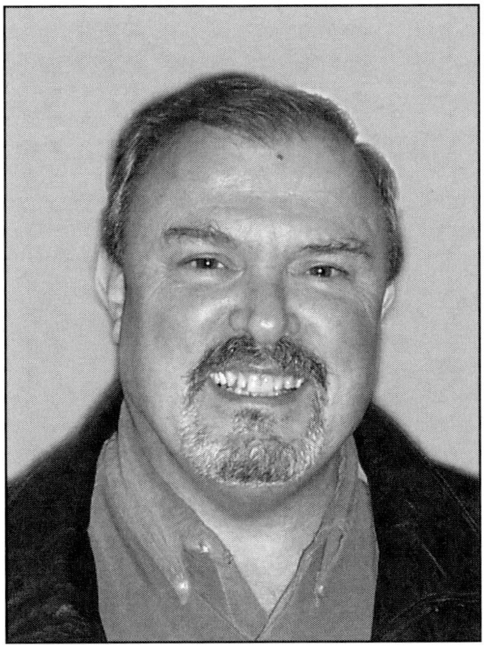

Cram received a Biomedical Equipment Technology degree from Texas State Technical Institute (now Texas State Technical College Waco) and worked as a biomedical technician while completing his Bachelor and Master of Science degrees in Biomedical Engineering from Texas A&M University. He has published extensively on topics relating to the biomedical and biotechnology fields in addition to being an editor of *The Journal of Clinical Engineering* for the past eight years. An instructor at TSTC Waco from 2004-07, Cram also developed the school's new biotechnology program. He currently serves as President of Dominion Biomedical in College Station, Texas.

Selby Holder

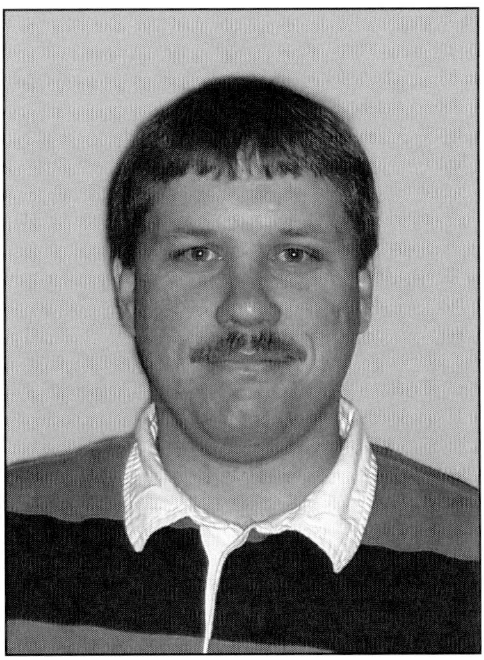

Holder graduated from Connally High School in Waco, Texas, with honors in 1989 and only a year later graduated from Texas State Technical Institute (now Texas State Technical College Waco) with a Biomedical Equipment Technology degree. He was subsequently employed by Healthcare Biomedical Services of Waco for eleven years and worked on a variety of medical devices including defibrillators, monitors, diagnostic ultrasounds, sterilizers, infusion devices, and more. Since 1999 he has been a certified biomedical technician. After the birth of his son—and therefore wanting to spend more time at home than on the road—Holder became an instructor at TSTC Waco in 2002. Currently, he serves as Cluster Director for the Electrical/Electronics Core.

TSTC Publishing

Established in 2004, TSTC Publishing is a provider of high-end technical instructional materials and related information to institutions of higher education and private industry. "High end" refers simultaneously to the information delivered, the various delivery formats of that information, and the marketing of materials produced. More information about the products and services offered by TSTC Publishing may be found at its Web site: http://publishing.tstc.edu/.

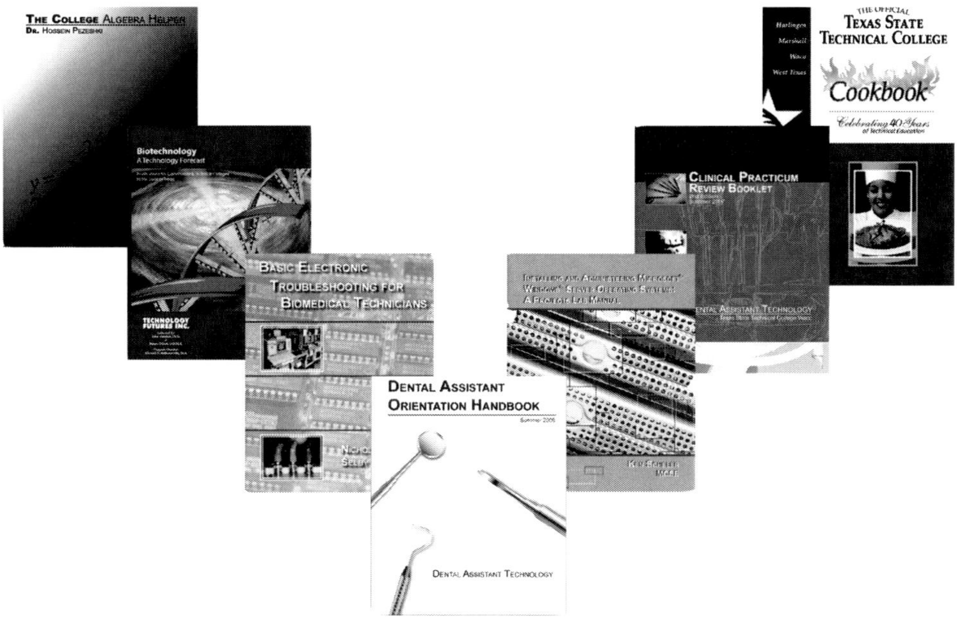